TESTIMONIALS OF HEALING

"Dr Reilly saved me when I had three herniated discs and I couldn't stand up straight. He combined a series of different modalities and saved me from having surgery. He listens well, very attentive, supportive and caring. His office staff always greet you with warm friendly smiles and are really welcoming too."

—ALISON J., RN

"I had constant headaches from the back of my shoulders to the top of my head for three years. I was taking 6-8 pain pills a day. My blood pressure was high and wouldn't go lower even though they tried six different medications. I saw an orthopedic specialist and internist and tried drugs and physical therapy without relief. Dr Reilly found my problem right away. My headaches were gone in two weeks and my blood pressure is back to normal. Please don't put off going for help! Doc Reilly has been a miracle to me."

—JOANN L.

"I had neck, shoulder and arm pain for four months. Drugs gave temporary relief. I feel like a new person, not being in any pain after one treatment."

—VIOLA T.

"Dr. Reilly, how can I thank you enough for all you have done, and continue to do, for me. It is such a relief to know that I can live pain-free by getting regular chiropractic adjustments. I remember when I first came to you -- it must be 9 years ago by now -- I was in chronic pain. Unfamiliar with chiropractic at that time, I was initially apprehensive but you helped me feel at ease right away and within a few short weeks, I was pain-free. What a relief!

With the chronic condition that I have, I know that periodic adjustments are necessary to maintain pain-free living and I am so grateful that I can count on you to help me with the chiropractic care that I need to live life more fully. I always feel so much better after receiving an adjustment.

Over the years I have experienced and seen how dedicated and genuinely concerned you are for the health and wellbeing of your patients. I also admire how you are always the first doctor of chiropractic in the area to research and embrace state-of-the-art technologies that enhance the health of your clients. Your generosity for giving back to the community with various fundraisers, donations and sponsorships is yet another testament to your compassion and kindness. It is no wonder that you have been awarded the prestigious Doctor of the Year award.

You are so kind and compassionate and I admire and appreciate your medical and technical expertise as well. I sincerely appreciate everything you have done to help me have a better quality of life and I thank you from the bottom of my heart."

—RAIN

"I had severe neck pain, fibromyalgia, headaches, leg pain and restless leg syndrome. I tried medications; physical therapy and massage therapy some only gave temporary relief. Now my neck pain, headaches and leg pain are gone. Try chiropractic, the results are wonderful. I have not felt this good in years."

—A. OWENS

"I had chronic pain due to; Fibromyalgia, migraines and arthritis for over ten years. I tried physical therapy, saw orthopedists and rheumatologists and was in and out of hospitals. I was taking a long list of medications. Today I am pain free and off almost all my medication. I have more energy and feel like I got my life back. Dr. Reilly worked like nothing else ever had."

—TRACY R.

"A neurosurgeon diagnosed me with three ruptured discs, degenerative disc disease, and arthritis and hip trouble. I was told surgery would not help and I would have to live with the pain. I tried physical therapy, drugs, painful back injections, acupuncture, pool therapy, thirty traction treatments and other chiropractors with little relief. I spent eight months in bed. I couldn't move or turn over without screaming in pain. Since going to Dr Reilly, I can sit comfortably, sleep at night and do things most of us take for granted. Dr Reilly cares about his patients, not their money. Dr Reilly is the best; if you are in pain give Dr Reilly a chance."

—CLIFF D.

"I had low back and hip pain for three years. I had an MRI, saw an orthopedic surgeon and tried physical therapy. Through Dr Reilly's knowledge, expertise and devotion to helping and healing his fellow human beings, I have received some of the best care imaginable by a doctor. For the excellent physical care and healing, the kindness, patience and understanding, I am truly grateful to Dr Reilly and his staff."

—PATRICIA M.

"I have had neck and low back pain, sciatica and headaches for nineteen years. Traveling in my car was almost impossible. An orthopedic surgeon diagnosed me with degenerative disc disease. He said surgery was risky with no guarantee of success. He prescribed medications and physical therapy. After treatments at Fairview Chiropractic Center I began to regain mobility in my neck, had a decrease in my pain, headaches that are very much reduced and am more comfortable traveling. In addition to being a gifted chiropractor Dr Reilly is a compassionate man. If you or someone you know were suffering from similar conditions I would strongly recommend seeing Dr Reilly. I highly recommend him."

—ELLIE G.

"I had muscle spasms in my neck and low back for five months as a result of a car accident. I have been helped in every way. My back and neck no longer give me any problems."

—SARAH W.

"I had been in constant severe low back, hip and leg pain for five years. I could hardly walk and it affected my entire life. I had been to several orthopedic surgeons, I went to two years of physical therapy, numerous sessions with a pain management doctor, saw my family doctor, did lots of exercise and took lots of pain medications. Since coming to see Dr Reilly I am almost pain free and I can walk much better. If you are in any pain go see Dr Reilly first."

—LARRY JOE M.

"I could barely walk into your office. I had seen three other medical doctors without relief other than pain pills and they had no idea what was wrong with me. I had lived with hip pain for six weeks. Your treatment worked almost instantaneously. I am so excited just to walk without pain. I thank God for sending you to me; I am back to my normal life. You have worked miracles for me as far as I am concerned, Thank You!"

—NANCY A.

"I had low back pain, a pinched nerve, a bad disc and tight muscles for about a year. I was taking prescription pain medications. When I first came to see Dr Reilly I was walking with a four-point cane. He has helped me so much that I don't need to use it anymore. Dr Reilly treats his patients with kindness and he understands our problems."

—VIRGINIA M.

"I had neck/shoulder pain and migraines for years. I used prescription medications for relief. Don't wait so long to get help because it does work and you don't have to be in pain or take drugs for relief."

—DEBBIE O.

"I had neck and shoulder pain for several years. I saw an orthopedic surgeon who suggested surgery and other chiropractic care that was ineffective. I have been taught correct posture and am now basically free of pain. My neck is getting its curve back. Absolutely try chiropractic before you let your surgeon operate on you."

—DAUNE V., RN

"I had neck and shoulder pain and stiffness associated with ankylosing spondylitis for over twenty years. I had tried several MDs and was taking prescription anti-inflammatories. Chiropractic greatly helped, I'm taking almost no anti-inflammatories."

—ROBERT L.

"I had neck and shoulder pain for almost three years. I was using pain medications that put me to sleep. The first visit made me pain free. In addition to being pain free I haven't had any colds or sinus infections, my sleep has improved and my overall health is better."

—P.O.

"I had severe neck/shoulder pain and headaches for over 15 years. I tried everything else, muscle relaxants, pain relievers and cortisone injections with little relief. Now I can move my neck without pain, I don't wake up unable to turn without moving my entire body. It's worth giving chiropractic a try. It's nice not having the pain."

—CONNIE G.

"I had headaches, neck, shoulder and low back pain from an automobile accident. I saw an orthopedic surgeon. I tried medication and physical therapy without relief. My severe pain is gone and I'm still getting better. Don't put off going to a chiropractor, I have gotten wonderful care with Dr Reilly."

—PEGGY R.

"I had shoulder joint pain on and off for twenty years. I had x-rays and joint injections with dye without results. I have been helped through chiropractic adjustments and exercises. I absolutely recommend it."

—W.D. K.

"I came home from work and I literally could not walk, (I hobbled). I spent the weekend in bed. My mom and family physician Jeffrey Tait both told me to try your treatments, I admit I was skeptical. After you helped me out of the chair, I hobbled into your x-ray room. Thanks to you I walked out of your office. It's amazing how much better I felt in one visit. Shortly I was on my way to being 100%. I recommend you to everyone I know. Thanks"

—DENISE K.

"I have shoulder, hip and back pain that got worse after driving for almost ten years. I tried celebrex, ibuprofen, physical therapy and other chiropractic treatments. Dr Reilly has helped me quite a bit more than medical doctors, physical therapists or other chiropractors."

—FRED S.

"I had a lot of pain in my back and hips for years with no easing. I tried drugs and physical therapy, they did not work. I doubted chiropractic could help me. I had been told a lot of foolish things. I got a lot of relief after coming to see Dr Reilly. After a few visits I felt great. Don't wait, the sooner you get started and stay with it the better off you'll be. You wont believe the difference."

—RUTH R.

GETTING THE HEALTH YOU DESERVE NOW!

GETTING THE HEALTH YOU DESERVE NOW!

NEW HOPE FOR CHRONIC ILLNESS WITH NEUROMETABOLIC THERAPY

DR. EDWARD G. REILLY , D.C.

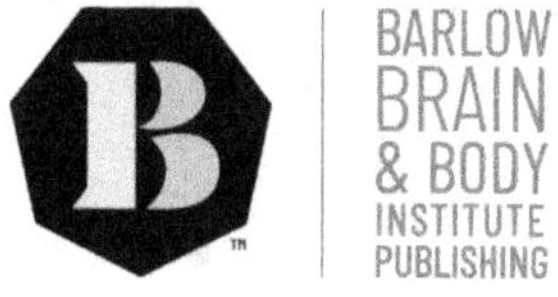

BARLOW
BRAIN
& BODY
INSTITUTE
PUBLISHING

Barlow Brain & Body Institute
266 County Road 506
Shannon, MS 38868
www.barlowbrainandbody.com

I want to thank my father, Bill Reilly, for being a great light in the world to me, my family; those whose lives he helped, and those he touched. He spent 40 years running into burning buildings while everyone else was running out. Next to my mom, Geri, the best mother in the world, I would also like to thank my brothers and sisters; nieces and nephews; Granny Taylor; my loving wife, Adina, who we lost much too soon; my amazing children, Connor and Leia; and my sweet Elizabeth.

Thanks to my brother Bill who introduced me to chiropractic and kicked me onto this road when I was training for the NYC marathon, as to how chiropractic could be my purpose.

To Dr. Andy Barflow, a visionary healer and teacher and mentor. And the many teachers and to the nearly 15,000 patients who let me touch their lives and learn from them and many, many others along the way…and God.

TABLE OF CONTENTS

FOREWORD

In today's fast-paced world, it is all too common for us to
neglect our health and well-being. We often find ourselves
caught up in the chaos of everyday life, barely giving our
bodies and minds the attention they deserve. However, there is
hope. In the midst of this whirlwind, Dr. Ed Reilly's ground-
breaking book, "Getting the Health You Deserve Now," illumi-
nates a path towards true wellness and vitality.

Drawing from his extensive knowledge and experience in
the field of healing, Dr. Reilly unveils the fundamental prin-
ciples that unlock the body's innate ability to heal itself. With
a compassionate and insightful approach, "Getting the Health
You Deserve Now" takes readers on a transformative journey,
guiding them to untangle the intricate web of dysfunction that
often impedes recovery.

What sets this book apart is Dr. Reilly's practical and action-
able guidance, making it accessible to anyone seeking to improve
their health. By addressing key areas such as optimizing oxygen

and glucose levels, stimulating neurological pathways, and addressing autoimmune diseases, readers are empowered to take control of their well-being and enact positive changes.

Moreover, Dr. Reilly delves into the detrimental effects of inflammation, the often-overlooked issue of neurotoxicity, and the significance of gut health. By shedding light on these crucial aspects, he equips readers with the knowledge needed to overcome long-standing health problems that may have eluded explanation.

If you or a loved one are grappling with a mysterious health issue, "Getting the Health You Deserve Now" is an essential read. Dr. Reilly's compassionate and insightful guidance not only deepens understanding of your condition but also offers practical solutions that can transform lives. Within the pages of this book lies the power to make a difference.

Remember, the right decision can change everything. By embarking on this journey of achieving optimal health, you are taking a transformative step towards a healthier, happier, and more vibrant life. Let Dr. Ed Reilly be your trusted guide as you unlock the secrets to the health you deserve.

Wishing you renewed health and vitality,

DR. ANDY BARLOW, DC
Founder of the Barlow Brain and Body Institute
Graduate of both the Carrick Institute of Functional
Neurology and American College of Functional Neurology

PART ONE

SHARED PHILOSOPHY

CHAPTER 1

FOLLOWING MY PURPOSE—EVEN THOUGH I THOUGHT I WAS ...

I didn't always know that I wanted to become a chiropractor. I was very much into natural health, lots of running, biking, swimming, diet, and nutrition. I was living a great life working in a corporate position at AT&T with people from all over the world on my team. I was in the management development program where I completed my executive MBA degree, grateful that it was paid for and that I was on a career path that could have led to senior vice president in the company. I thought I was happy; I was not looking for a career change by any means.

In 1982, I planned to run in the New York City Marathon. I was training for about six-to-eight months and noticed a growing pain from my lower back into my right leg about six weeks before the marathon. After going to my family doctor, my prognosis was bleak. He advised I had developed sciatica, started me on some medication, and booked my physical therapy appointments. They both said it was time for me to stop running. In no way, shape, or form would I be able to run the marathon safely.

Luckily for me, my brother was in chiropractic school at the time. When I told him that I would not be able to run, he suggested I see a local sports chiropractor. My first response was to let him know I had already been to a doctor and a physical therapist and that I had sciatica—in case he did not hear me the first time. He repeated that I should give it a try. I gave in and decided I had nothing to lose, so I made the appointment.

I told the chiropractor, "Look, I do not think you can help me. I have been to the doctor and a physical therapist, and they both said I must stop running." But the chiropractor accepted me as a patient and started working with me. Within two weeks, I was able to run without any pain. This experience led me to an epiphany that the traditional l medical model does not have the whole picture. I was shocked that a chiropractor could help with sciatica when a doctor and a physical therapist could not! I was so grateful that I got to run the marathon after all.

This experience led me to co-create my booklet, "What to Do When Traditional Medicine Fails" last year, and I am writing this book to go into further detail.

Training for the NYC Marathon 10 years later, a similar situation occurred. I was training for about six months. Eight weeks out from the marathon, I developed severe Achilles tendonitis. I was in a lot of pain and taking ibuprofen to go on training runs. When I could not run any further, I went back to my medical doctor and the same advice came rolling in: Take medicine, go to see a foot doctor, another series of physical therapy sessions, and whatever you do, stop running. Again, I felt defeated. I had been training for so long, and these doctors were experts who were trying to help me. But, out of desperation, I talked with my brother Bill, and moaned that I would not be running the marathon. He said, "Why don't you see the sports medicine chiropractor who helped you with your sciatica years ago?"

I proceeded to ask him, why would I go to a chiropractor for a for a foot problem?

I have already been to a foot expert.

"Chiropractors only work on backs" But I was desperate, so even though I was not sure what he could do, I went. And just like before, he started working on my foot and I was back to running in two weeks. It reinforced that earlier thought: Traditional medical doctors do not know everything!

As I started to reflect on other experiences with traditional medical doctors, it brought me to my childhood experience with a ruptured appendix that everybody missed until I was near death. The best in medicine missed that. How does that happen? Thousands of people die every year from misdiagnosed appendicitis. Another 500,000+ die annually from taking over-the-counter pain medications.

One morning in 1989, I was sitting at my desk in my office. This immediate thought just filled my brain. It was my first experience with a spiritual epiphany, along with meeting friends of Bill Wilson. I started the process of turning my life over completely to God.

I heard Christ, "You need to change the course of your life. You are not doing the right thing. What you are doing is good, but it does not bring meaning to your life. You are supposed to be helping others. You have a good job, but your purpose is in a different direction."

I was a single 33 year old. My first thought was, "I do not want to quit my job. I am not interested in a career change. I am set."

The response was, "Okay, but if you don't, you're going to regret it because this is what you're supposed to be doing."

In frustration I thought, "Leave me alone! I am not quitting. I am not going back to school." Nothing about this conversation in my head made sense. But it would not go away. Instead, it continued to get louder.

And every day for the next two years I felt unsettled. I did not want to live a life filled with regret, but I did not understand what I was supposed to do instead, so I prayed on that message while not really making any significant changes. I knew I had to figure out how I was going to follow the call and help people in a more meaningful way. I liked the idea of chiropractic school, but there was still a part of me that felt like it was kind of "quacky."

I investigated medical school, dental school, and a psychology doctorate. I thought back to the medical doctors who could not help when I went to them about my issues while training for marathons. I felt inspired by my brother's chiropractic practice again. Then those thoughts started again, asking me to look at my experience with a chiropractor and how he could help me when it felt like no one else could. So I surrendered to the process and thought, "Okay, I will go back to school for six years and become a chiropractor."

After two years of ongoing contemplation, I sold my house and moved into a small apartment in Atlanta. I felt that I was on the verge of a complete do-over in my life. I sold everything I owned in preparation for making a move and never going back. Half of my friends said, "You're out of your mind." The other half said, "That's a lot of courage." There were days when I was not sure who I agreed with more, but I knew beyond a shadow of a doubt that I was called to do this work, and I was along for the ride.

I had my plan and put in my notice at AT&T in 1992. The company graciously gave me a four-year leave of absence so I could come back after finishing graduate school in Atlanta. I was still on the payroll and had all my health and dental insurance covered during that time. A few months before I graduated in 1996, the HR department called me to let me know that the following Monday would be the last day of my four-year leave, and if I did not go back to New Jersey, they would need to eliminate my position.

I was floored when I asked what would happen if I came up there on Monday, and they said they would lay me off and give me a severance check, along with one more year until the benefits ran out. I was excited to use that money towards my own practice one day.

At graduate school, there were some dark nights of the soul. My old life was gone and I was on what turned out to be a spiritual journey that gave me the life God wanted me to have. I would look around and ask myself, "What have I done?" I had a house and a great job from which I had just got up and left. And there I was, in a tiny apartment, going to classes and studying all the time. The process changed me. Not only did I learn how to be a chiropractor, but I also went through a series of epiphanies that changed me as a human being for the better. I had so much more knowledge and a lot of knowingness—not "thinkingness"—that I was exactly where I was supposed to be. It led to meeting my beautiful, loving wife, Adina, starting a practice in Asheville, and raising a family, Connor and Leia, in a beautiful mountain community.

Initially I started working with my brother in his practice in Hershey, Pennsylvania, for a part of 1997. I married Adina while she was finishing up her own chiropractic degree and I moved back to Atlanta so she could finish school. In January 1998, I worked in a clinic in Atlanta while my wife completed her coursework. We were debating moving back to New Jersey or finding a place in Asheville, North Carolina.

We were at the airport on our way to sign for a new office lease in New Jersey when a blizzard came in, stranding us at

Newark airport and missing our lease signing appointment. Sitting in the airport, we looked at each other and knew we would never sign that lease. It was serendipitous! Upon reflection, it was really God helping us make the right decision. It gave us a moment to pause and really consider what we wanted. Within three months, we had opened a practice in Asheville, and we had our first child six months into our new practice. At that time Adina and I opted for her to be a stay-at-home mom, which turned out to be the best decision she ever made. Thank you, God.

I could not have lived such a joyful life without making the choice to burn the proverbial ships and take the leap of faith. It was amazing to see all the things that fell into place! I met the love of my life while at graduate school, had two amazing children, Connor and Leia, which would never have happened if I had tried to hush that little voice and stay in my corporate job.

I was blessed to be able to live a purposeful life helping others and living my best life.

THE BELIEFS THAT DRIVE ME

Never Stop Learning!

I DO NOT WANT TO BE A CHIROPRACTIC NEURO METABOLIC EXPERT

I think it goes back to the epiphany I had. Every time I felt myself getting a bit lax, I would get that nudge again. "Hey, read this book. Go to this seminar. Meet with this person." And I keep moving forward. I am always looking for ways to improve, and to gain new knowledge that will continue to help people in new ways. I have completed nearly 4000 hours in post-doctoral training, I teach other doctors, have multiple advanced credentialing and am currently finishing a functional neurology teaching fellowship.

My belief is that there is an optimal health paradigm for humans. It's really about optimal communications within the body that lead to optimal health. Each system is neurologically dependent on another for health. Small changes in the level of sodium potassium in your blood can affect communications in all 70 trillion cells in your body negatively.

OPTIMAL HEALTH PARADIGM

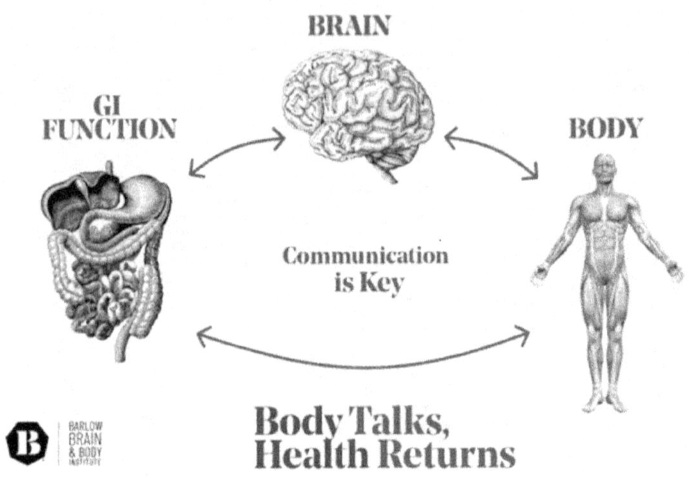

Where Are Your Blinky Lights?

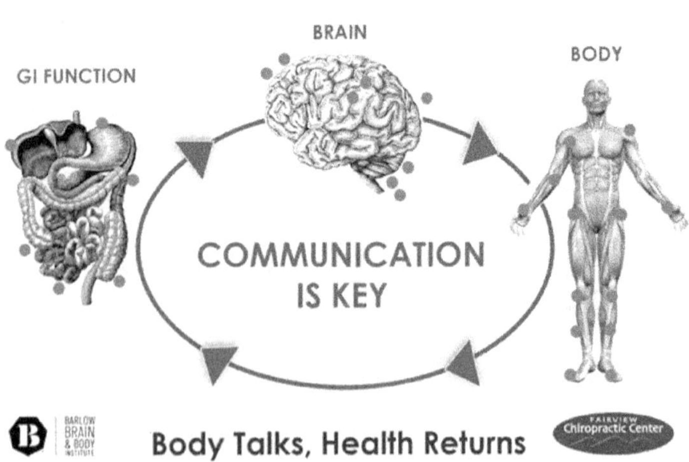

BLINKY LIGHTS

"Blinky lights" in the human body, detected through advanced testing, show up as seemingly unrelated factors, that when viewed by an expert can predict why someone has a complex health condition. These "blinky lights" are mostly not tested for or missed with traditional medical care.

Variations in blood sugar start inflammation in the entire body, damaging the most vulnerable tissue first: nerves, joints, internal organs, skin. High levels of C-reactive protein and homocysteine show systemic inflammation going on throughout the body, again targeting the most vulnerable tissues: nerves, joints, internal organs, skin. Gluten and other food sensitivities can lead to a breakdown of the intestinal lining, leading to leaky gut, systemic inflammation, and autoimmune disorders. Infections such as dental issues and Lyme disease can lay hidden, and are often underlying complex problems. Chronic mold exposure and toxic chemical exposure can't be ruled out, nor can underlying genetics. These are "blinky lights".

When the communications within the body break down, "blinky lights" show up in the body. The early warning signals are usually missed because of medical specialization. It's not the doctors' fault; our medical system has rigid approaches to helping people with chronic problems. They are becoming more and more narrowly focused and more often than not, they miss the big picture as shown in the diagram below.

Medicine has become very specialized today. This extreme specialization has led to a standard of care approach to complex health conditions. In effect, each specialist looks for health problems only within their specialty. I call it "blinky light doctoring."

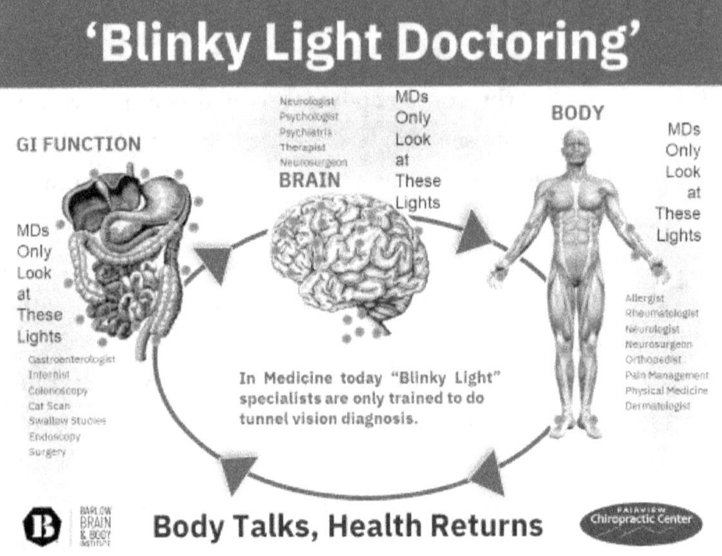

How can I be the best at helping others?

My wife passed away in 2019 after we went through a six-year-long medical trial. Cancer is a ruthless disease.

My mother is in stage five dementia. I am having those conversations with my family about whose turn it is to stay over, take her to the doctor, or get the groceries. I wish I had known five years ago that dementia can be helped with cutting edge testing, treatments, lifestyle, and diet modifications.

It makes me wonder what would happen if I had the ability to look at someone and find out that they have 10, 20 or 30 "blinky lights" that create whole body inflammation which increases the predisposition for any chronic illness. Cancer, autoimmune disorders, and chronic health problems are all made worse with systemic inflammation. Can reducing systemic inflammation help with the progression of chronic health conditions? I think the answer is yes.

And when looking at dementia, traditional medicine is looking for just one drug to treat every person. But there are many "blinky lights" that get missed. What if we could identify all of them and help the brain, body and GI function to begin healing before they go into those deeper disease stages?

As an example of this notion of "blinky lights," science has identified 36 factors that lead to the process of developing dementia. Medicine has spent billions in research looking for the single cause of dementia; in fact over 2000 clinical trials have failed to produce any one drug that can address the progression of dementia. It is time to use the cutting edge testing and treatments that have been shown to help in published medical journals. One study showed a reversal of Alzheimer's **WITHOUT the use of drugs.** In that study, natural protocols were used to address the BODY BRAIN AND GI dysfunction. Science has found the "blinky lights" of dementia in the body and GI tract as well as the brain. This is where I think research should be focused, not on a single cure. It doesn't exist because there isn't one cause.

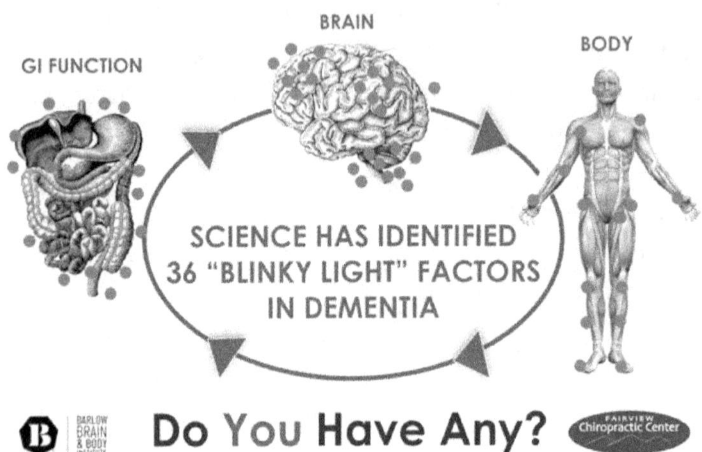

I love to help people by being proactive with their body systems instead of being reactive after the fact. I started out wanting to help people with sciatica or foot or neck problems the way a DC helped me. But it turned into a relentless quest to help each person who comes through my door to alter how their life looks and make it better because they met me. I now try to help the whole human and not just the spot that hurts.

Follow your convictions.

If you are getting a nagging feeling that you need to make an appointment with your local chiropractor, follow that lead. Or, if you keep hearing that it is time to make significant changes, take the leap of faith and see where the journey takes you.

Maybe this book is your "nudge," like I got to go to chiropractic school, to seek out help for a problem you have just been living with, or after being told there is nothing that can be done.

I am living a complete life.

It is incredible to think of all the things that happened once I surrendered to my purpose. I met an amazing woman; we opened our practice in the beautiful city of Asheville; we raised two exceptional children and I am blessed to do what I love!

We may be able to help you, but you have a role to play.

I am a doctor, but my role is also as a teacher. I have delivered over 3000 public health lectures for patients and other doctors. I have trained other doctors to do the kind of work I do. And with any teacher/student relationship, we are here together as a collaboration. We both must put in the work so you can have a better life that ripples out to your loved ones for generations to come.

I understand how difficult it can be to make major changes to your life, but I can tell you from experience that it is worth it in the end.

It is about optimizing recovery by starting where you are at.

It is not about just living longer. It is about living the best life longer. I want to live a full life, and that is what I want for the people I help. In order to live your best life, we will work together to create normal communication throughout your body's systems and eliminate your "blinky lights.".

The philosophy is to find the problem within the human body and look for the "blinking lights" that indicate which systems in the body are asking for help. I can then help connect the dots within their human system health concerns and create the best program for you to help your body communicate the way it was meant to all along.

CHAPTER 3

THERE'S MORE BELOW THE SURFACE

TIP OF THE ICEBERG

Have you ever studied a diagram of an iceberg? From above the surface of the water, your eye can only see about 10% of the iceberg's total mass while the remaining 90% remains out of sight, lurking below the surface. An iceberg is a good metaphor for the way we should understand the total picture of our health. The symptoms we experience represent only 10-15% of the issue that is causing those obvious symptoms to appear. To understand the whole picture, uncover the web of dysfunction, and discover the path to true healing, we have to delve below the surface.

Symptoms can also be compared to the check engine light on your car. If you're on a road trip and the check engine light comes on, you're alerted to a problem with your vehicle. Would taking a piece of duct tape and covering up that check engine light solve the problem? Absolutely not, it would only prevent you from seeing the blinking light that's alerting you to a bigger issue. In fact, covering up the check engine light puts you in greater danger in the long run because what started out as a small problem will get worse and worse if you continue on your road trip and don't address the problem. Pretty soon, you're sitting on the side of the road with smoke and steam rolling out of your engine. This is what it's like when we take medication to mask our symptoms. Covering them up doesn't change the fact that there's a problem. To really figure out the issue with our car, we must go to a mechanic and have them look under the hood. To figure out the issue with our body, we need to untangle the web of dysfunction that's causing the symptom to surface.

In a car, there are a multitude of reasons why the check engine light appears. It could be a fuel issue, a spark plug issue, a battery issue, or something else entirely. Think of your health symptoms as your body's check engine light. In the same way that a check engine light comes on for a variety of reasons, our symptoms can result from a variety of health issues. This is one of the most important concepts that I teach my patients - the root cause of symptoms is different for every single person because their web of dysfunction is completely unique.

There are three main reasons why a "one size fits all" strategy does not work for solving chronic health problems. The first reason is that two people could be experiencing the same exact symptoms for completely different reasons. For example, numbness, tingling or burning of the feet can be caused by nerve damage in the lumbar spine at the L5 vertebrae. However, it can also be caused by Type 2 diabetes or anemia. All three disorders can cause the exact same symptom for totally different reasons. To make the tangled web of dysfunction even more complicated, many of my patients have more than one root cause of their symptoms. The bottom line is that every person's health issues must be treated uniquely.

The second reason why a "one size fits all" approach doesn't work is because a doctor with preconceived notions tends to miss important clues that reveal what's really going on beneath the surface. For someone with chronic health problems, there are multiple mechanisms that can go awry and cause dysfunction, yet show up as the same kind of symptom. These mechanisms include elements like blood sugar, anemia, or destruction of the neurological pathways. If the root cause is never addressed, the correct mechanism that needs restoration and healing will never be found. Each person is a custom case. As a functional neuro-metabolic doctor, it's my job to be smart enough to look below the surface and examine the 90% that's beneath the surface.

The third reason why a "one size fits all approach" does not work for solving chronic health problems is because it tends to produce doctors that are symptom-reduction oriented rather than results oriented. As a functional neuro-medicine doctor, I want my patients to actually get better. Every time I walk into a room with a patient, I check my ego at the door because I want to solve their problems, not mask them. I am result oriented, and I am solution oriented. I'm committed to getting results for my patients, and I will exhaust all of my resources to do it. I treat each patient like a custom, one-of-a-kind 10,000 piece puzzle. When I accept a patient for care, we sit down together and start working on that puzzle until we uncover the root cause(s) and form a plan to heal them. To truly heal, we need to target and solve the core problem. We must untangle the neuro-metabolic web of dysfunction and start a journey to regeneration and wellness.

With the first three chapters as our foundation, let's go deeper by defining and then explaining the Seven Keys to healing your chronic health problems.

PART TWO

SHARED UNDERSTANDING

CHAPTER 4

UNTANGLING THE WEB OF DYSFUNCTION

There are seven key areas of health that I look at when I'm trying to untangle someone's web of dysfunction. Depending on how they're treated, these seven keys can either foster wellness and longevity or create debilitating chronic health problems because each of these keys either adds to our health or actively takes away and destroys our health. Throughout my years of practice and study, I've discovered that any kind of disruption in these seven areas is going to cause disconnection and dysfunction (check engine light) which may eventually turn into chronic issues. When I work with a patient to help them with their chronic health problems, this is always where we begin. When these seven areas are treated well, it unleashes your body's superpower which is its ability to heal itself.

THE SEVEN KEYS

1. Oxygen: Number One of the BIG Three. It is necessary and essential for life. Anoxia (which means "without oxygen") equals death. The brain and nervous system need three elements to function at peak level, and oxygen is one of them. Oxygen is the deal breaker when it comes to neurological health. The less oxygen we have in our

bodies, the more things start to malfunction and the less capacity our bodies have to heal themselves.

2. Glucose: Number Two of the BIG Three. Glucose is your blood sugar. It's the fuel that your body needs in order to heal itself. It's also needed for the nervous system to self-regulate and function optimally. A good metaphor is that it's like the gasoline for your car engine. Cars run at a certain octane level, and if that level gets out of balance, the car isn't going to run properly. Our bodies work the same way with glucose. If there's too little, it can't function at its optimal level. If there's too much, it's not good for optimal performance either.

3. Stimulation: Number Three of the BIG Three. Stimulation is one of the main three things that the nervous system needs in order to function. The importance of stimulation can't be overstated. As Einstein once said, "Nothing happens until something moves," and in the body, no healing happens until something is stimulated. Without stimulation, the body's systems will weaken and fail. With proper stimulation, those systems will thrive and remain strong.

4. Autoimmune Disorders: Autoimmune disorders are kind of like "friendly fire." They develop when our immune system starts attacking itself instead of a foreign invader. Our immune systems should only kill the "bad guys" like viruses, but when it starts to malfunction, it doesn't just destroy antigens, it also attacks our own tissues.

5. Inflammation: Logic tells you that if your house was on fire, you wouldn't start rebuilding it until after the blazes were put out. Inflammation is like a fire in your body, and it can't start to heal until that fire is gone. True healing cannot take place until your body's inflammation is reduced.

6. Neurotoxins: These toxins are anything that's taken into the body that causes neurological damage. Unfortunately neurotoxins are much more common than you may imagine. Table sugar is a neurotoxin. High fructose corn syrup is a neurotoxin. The artificial sweetener Aspartame is a neurotoxin. Drinking water out of a disposable plastic bottle is neurotoxic. We'll talk more in upcoming chapters about how to eliminate these harmful toxins from your life.

7. Gut Health: The role of gut health is paramount because poor gut health is a trigger for autoimmune conditions and out of control inflammatory responses. We must heal our guts in order to heal our brains and bodies. If you have a bad brain, you're guaranteed to have a bad gut too. We must restore optimal gut health and reconnect the gut-brain axis in order to achieve true healing.

While each of these seven areas are important to address individually, their true power for healing comes alive when we realize that all of these elements are interconnected. Gut health and autoimmune conditions are connected. Neurotoxins and inflammation are linked. Oxygen and stimulation are crucial to one another's roles. The body is a holistic system that must be in homeostasis in order to heal itself and function optimally. By keeping these seven primary keys in focus, your health can transform from symptom mitigation to a state of true healing and regeneration. Now that we've looked at an overview of the seven keys to optimal health, let's break each key down in greater detail.

CHAPTER 5

KEY 1 – OXYGEN

THE ROLE OF OXYGEN

Oxygen is essential for life. This element, which makes up about 21% of the earth's atmosphere at sea level, is key to our health because our bodies need it in order to function on a cellular level. We can go without food almost forty days, and we can last about four days without water. However, we can only survive for approximately four minutes without oxygen. If the brain is deprived of oxygen for longer than that, it's a recipe for severe neurological damage and even death. Our cells need oxygen in order to make ATP, which is essentially the "energy" on which our bodies run. If there isn't adequate energy, then the neurons (the cells responsible for receiving sensory input from the outside world and for sending motor commands to our muscles) fail and many forms of neurological dysfunction and chronic health problems may follow.

Oxygen deprivation isn't only a reality for people who need to be "on oxygen" or are constantly hooked up to a machine. In fact, I see many, many patients who are lacking oxygen because they're anemic. An anemic person may have decreased blood circulation issues which equals decreased oxygen to the tissues of the body. Many of my patients have been anemic for years but no doctor has taken the time to explain to them what that means for their health so they don't understand the full implications of that diagnosis.

Our bodies must have an adequate supply of oxygen in order to heal, especially when it comes to chronic health problems. Oxygen plays a crucial role in helping us heal from chronic health issues because of something called "resting membrane potential of the nerve cells." When a nerve is asked to perform a task but it's lacking oxygen, it's similar to an empty soap dispenser. You can pump and pump but nothing is going to happen. On the contrary, when the dispenser is full, it may be so primed that soap is coming out without any pumping. In the same way, oxygen impacts the nervous system's ability to function because it's what "primes the pump" for the nerve cells and gives it the energy to do its job.

The nervous system is made up of individual cells called neurons, and to maintain the health of these neurons, oxygen is crucial. Healthy neurons and an optimally functioning nervous system are essential building blocks for structural integrity of the cells, fighting chronic health issues and healing the body. Let's take a moment to dive deeper into understanding neurons and their function in our bodies.

A neuron's job is to transmit communication from the brain to the body and from the body back to the brain. Neurons communicate in two ways: electronically (similar to the electrical system in your home) and chemically (called neurotransmitters). In order for neurons to optimize communication between the brain and the body (and vice versa), they need three things: oxygen, glucose, and stimulation. If any of one of those three elements are taken away, you get neurons that don't "fire" properly, and malfunctioning neurons may cause brain fog, attention, memory issues as well as numbness, tingling and pins and needles sensation in the body.

If these neurons are interfered with, stunted, blunted or damaged in any way, the stage is set for an environment of dysfunction, which then may lead to a disease process.

To understand the disruptive effect of malfunctioning neurons, consider your home's internet connection. When the connection is interrupted or slowed, problems begin to appear. Your Netflix show appears grainy or your pictures don't download properly. Now think about your brain trying to communicate with all 75 trillion cells in your body. Imagine how easily things could go awry in that kind of system. So it is with our bodies and the complex wonder that is our neurological system. If the neurons that comprise our neurological system don't have an adequate supply of oxygen, the body can't heal itself properly because its main communication system is compromised.

There are a few ways to discover if you are oxygen deficient or not. To test a patient's oxygen levels at the clinic, I use a tool called a pulse oximeter. It's put on the tip of the finger and measures oxygen levels. Another way to test oxygen levels is by taking a person's blood pressure. If it's too low, it means the tissues of the body are not getting enough blood supply, and blood is what transports oxygen within the body. The third way to test oxygen levels is through blood work. I look at the total red blood cell count, and if that's too low, it's a sign of oxygen deficiency. These measurement tools are used to see how oxygen deficient someone may be and helps me determine how to treat them best. Signs of poor circulation are cold hands, cold feet, white fingernails (should be pink in color), and nail fungus. There's a saying in functional neurology, "cold hands, cold feet equals cold brain." Meaning, if you have poor circulation in your hands and feet, you probably have poor circulation in your brain as well.

RESULTS FROM OXYGEN

In order to understand how important oxygen is for healing chronic health problems, the main thing to grasp is that a person's oxygen level determines how much stimulation can be put into their nervous system before it "fails" (aka ceases to properly relay the stimulation). This system failure is known as "exceeding metabolic capacity" or EMC. At that point, the nervous system can take no more stimulation and may react with a headache, dizziness, or equilibrium problems.

If you're suffering from anemia, the first thing you may experience is a lack of concentration, focus, and attention. This may eventually turn into memory loss and dementia, but if you catch it early enough, it may be reversed. Lack of oxygen may also cause your extremities to change color, your nails to turn white, or you may lack hair on your lower extremities.

When your body is deficient of oxygen, many internal systems begin to misfire and go awry. The signals traveling from the body to your brain travel at roughly 270 mph. If there's a lack of oxygen, those major neural pathways become compromised and can't convey those fast-moving signals. If your oxygen level is skewed at all, it can lead to numbness, tingling, sensations of pins and needles, and other strange symptoms that show the neurons are misfiring.

There are a few simple, at-home tests you can do to see if you are anemic, aka lacking oxygen and lack of circulation. Start by looking at your fingernails. Are they pink? (Pink is good.) Or are they white? (White is bad.) What color are your toes? Are they blue? (Blue is bad.) Or purple? (Purple very bad.) You can also check for "pitting edema." If you push your finger into your lower leg and it doesn't rebound quickly, you are likely anemic. Toe fungus is another clue that you're not getting enough oxygen to your extremities, or if you always have cold fingers and toes (or cold extremities in general) that's a sign of anemia and poor circulation.

Bloodwork is also a great way to tell if you're lacking oxygen. If you've had blood tests in the last six months, examine your results to see if your red blood cell (RBC) count is low. If it is, that's a clue. If your hemoglobin (HGB) is too low, you are anemic. If you have low hematocrit (HCT) that's also an indicator of anemia. Your blood is like the 18-wheeler that delivers oxygen to your body's tissues, so those numbers are solid indicators of whether you're getting adequate oxygen supply or not.

If you suspect you are anemic, increasing the supply of oxygen to your body may impact your overall health in many positive ways. First of all, you'll notice an increase in energy and endurance and your mental endurance will also improve. You may also notice a better ability to focus for long periods of time. Many patients tell me they start sleeping better, feel better and have more mental clarity. All of these positive results start to happen because the neurons have enough oxygen to fire properly.

YOUR FIRST STEP

There are many simple ways to increase your oxygen levels. At the clinic, I often have anemic patients do exercise with oxygen therapy. They put an oxygen supply mask over their face and then ride a stationary bike for 15 minutes, called Exercise With Oxygen Therapy (EWOT). This is a very powerful therapy for oxygenating the body as well as the brain, because not only is oxygen being pumped through the mask, but the body and brain naturally increase their ability to receive oxygen as well as improve circulation when performing EWOT.

A few other simple strategies to increase oxygen levels include walking for at least thirty minutes per day and doing deep breathing exercises. Deep breathing or "forced breathing" exercises actually help stimulate the frontal lobe areas of your brain. The key to forced breathing is a 1:2 ratio. Start with breathing in deeply for four seconds and out for eight seconds, if you can perform this task move up to six seconds in and twelve seconds out. Optimal performance would be eight seconds in and sixteen seconds out. For chronic health suffers, eight in and sixteen out will be a challenge. These activities cause stimulation to the neurological pathways and inundate the body with oxygen. If you can't currently walk for thirty minutes, start by walking for five or six minutes per day. The most important thing is to stimulate the neurological system. Motion is life! Bicycling, either on a stationary bike or outdoors, is also excellent. Don't forget about swimming, it's low impact on your joints and very beneficial to your health. Take what you have at home and use it. It doesn't cost you anything to go outside and walk or do some forced breathing exercises.

When you go for your daily walk, swing your arms in an over exaggerated fashion. Non-linear complex movements (figure eight motions or writing your A,B,C's) will stimulate your cerebellum which in turn stimulates your brain. It's a win-win because it not only gets blood flowing to the extremity doing the non-linear movement, it also increases blood flow to the part of the cerebellum and brain which controls your extremities.

Now that we've covered the key health element of oxygen, let's look at the next key to improving chronic health problems.

CHAPTER 6

KEY 2 — GLUCOSE

THE ROLE OF GLUCOSE

You may have heard the word "glucose" before, but what exactly is it and why is it so important to our health? Glucose is simply our blood sugar, and it's the "fuel" that drives our nervous system. It plays an essential role in healing chronic problems because it supplies our nervous system with the energy it needs to do its job. Of course, healing only happens when our glucose is in optimal range (85-99) and when our A1C is below 5.6. Both of these numbers are a part of routine bloodwork.

In the same way that a car needs the proper fuel for its engine to start and to drive down the road, your nervous system needs the right levels of glucose to function optimally. Not only is the type of fuel important, the amount of fuel is key as well. If you don't have enough glucose, your body can't create the energy it needs to function. (Anything below 85 is hypoglycemia.) Yet if there's too much glucose present in your body, you'll feel slow, sluggish, and tired after eating. (Anything above 99 is hyperglycemia.) An abundance of glucose can also have a severely damaging effect on the nervous system. The higher the number, the more damaging the effects to your nervous system, brain, blood vessels and organs resulting in problems such as kidney failure or blindness.

There are a few ways to measure the glucose levels of your body. The first and most common way is through a simple blood test. Based on your results, you can see if your glucose (aka blood sugar) levels are too high or too low. The most simple, inexpensive (free!) at-home "test" to evaluate your glucose levels is to pay attention to the way you feel before and after meals.

If your blood sugar is too low (a condition known as "hypoglycemia"), you will feel a lack of concentration and focus as well as irritability prior to eating. Have you ever heard the term "hangry?" After you eat and your body becomes inundated with glucose, you'll start to feel better. If your glucose levels are too low, you may also have a tendency to wake up at night, have trouble sleeping, and often skip breakfast.

If your glucose levels are too high (known as "hyperglycemia"), you'll likely feel sleepy and sluggish after eating, especially if your meal contains lots of carbohydrates. Too much blood sugar may also cause you to be constantly thirsty, have headaches, or have trouble concentrating.

When your glucose levels are properly balanced, you don't experience the "hangry" feelings, the "crash" after a meal, or the constant cravings for sugars and starches. The only thing that should happen after you eat is that you feel full. That's it.

RESULTS FROM GLUCOSE

Let's dive deeper into what happens when you have a deficiency of glucose. The first symptoms of low blood sugar are the loss of focus, concentration, and attention. Many hypoglycemic people experience psychiatric symptoms like depression and anxiety, or they feel dizzy and have frequent headaches. These symptoms happen because the neurological system is lacking the fuel it needs to function properly. If glucose is the "fuel" that your nervous system needs to run on and the fuel gauge begins flashing "low," (there's that check engine light again) problems are going to surface. Essentially, your body's fuel source becomes so low that your neurons can't fire properly and begin losing function. Your car runs out of gas.

On the flip side, when there's an excess of glucose in the body, it's like taking sandpaper to the outside of an electrical cord. Inside the plastic sheath of the cord, there's a metal wire, which conducts electricity, just like our nervous system. If you take sandpaper to that coating and rub through the outer sheath, you can't put the protective sheath back on, leaving the bare wire exposed.

Too much glucose in the body has the same effect on the myelin sheath surrounding your nerve fibers. Myelin is an insulating layer that forms around nerves, including those in the brain and spinal cord. It is made up of protein and fatty substances, and it allows electrical impulses to transmit quickly and efficiently along the nerve cells. If that myelin coating is worn through, it can't be replaced as long as your glucose level is high. Once the nerve is exposed, the body's electrical system starts to malfunction because it lacks the protection it needs.

An excess of glucose can also cause balance problems, stability problems, coordination issues, and trouble with focus, attention, and concentration. Extreme cases of hyperglycemia can also cause kidney malfunction, blindness, or require the amputation of limbs. When there is too much glucose present in the bloodstream, things like insulin resistance start to appear, which is the precursor to diabetes. Interestingly enough, "Type 3" diabetes, a proposed term to describe the interlinked association between Type 1 and Type 2 diabetes and Alzheimer's disease, is also known as dementia and occurs when neurons in the brain become unable to respond to insulin, which is essential for basic tasks, including memory and learning.

Whether you are hypoglycemic (too little glucose) or hyperglycemic (too much glucose), the reality is that neither condition is ideal. Balanced, stable blood sugar levels are the goal, and when you get your glucose leveled out, everything begins to improve. You may even begin sleeping better because REM cycles are affected by both hyper and hypoglycemia. Your overall body function may improve, especially your liver, kidney, bladder and digestive health. How and why? Your organ system has to communicate with your brain and your brain has to communicate with your organs and it does this through the Vagus Nerve. With balanced blood sugar, you'll enjoy more energy and less mental and physical fatigue.

YOUR FIRST STEPS

When I see patients, I'm looking for an optimal fasting glucose level on their blood panel of anywhere from 85-99 and A1C below 5.6. This is different from the "medical normal" range which is 70-110. When I see a patient over 99, I consider them pre-diabetic because at this level, insulin resistance is already starting to destroy their nerve function, brain function, blood vessel function and organ function. When a person hits 126, they've officially entered into a disease process known as diabetes.

Anything below 85 is hypoglycemia meaning there's too little glucose in your blood for the neurological system to run at its peak level. If hypoglycemia gets to an advanced stage, it can actually cause you to pass out because there's such a severe lack of fuel that your neurons can't fire.

Your first step to balancing your blood sugar and stabilizing your glucose levels is to understand how and why you got to where you are today. Here's where I'm going to give you some tough love. Unless you are a Type 1 diabetic (which is an autoimmune disorder), this Type 2 diabetes is a self-inflicted condition. You did this to yourself. Ouch, I know that's hard to hear. The good news is that you can also undo it! This is where personal responsibility really comes into play.

To immediately begin stabilizing your glucose levels, I encourage you to start moving. Exercise burns off glucose, stimulates your nervous system, and increases your body's oxygen levels. Win, win, and win! Start with simple forms of movement like walking or bicycling, and then work up to more strenuous activities like swimming, workout classes, or weight lifting. Regardless of where you're at in your health journey, find a form of exercise that you enjoy and start doing it. Try to move your body every day. Again, motion is life! If you rest, you rust.

The second key to stabilizing your blood sugar is found in the kitchen. It's all about what you put in your mouth. What you put in your mouth is just as important as the way you move your body. Start tracking your food using a phone app like MyFitnessPal to find out how many grams of carbs and sugar you're consuming each day. You don't have to track your food forever, but committing to it for 60-90 days is one of the best tools to teach you how to eat properly. Most people are shocked when they see their initial numbers. Get rid of the bread, cake, and cookies. Eat less carbs and consume more healthy proteins and fats (baked chicken, fish, bison). Portion sizes are also crucial. Measure out your meals carefully and skip on seconds.

Glucose is essential for solving chronic health problems because it's the fuel that our neurological system needs to do its job. However, having too much or too little glucose can cause serious health issues and even create serious disease processes like diabetes. Doing these simple things can help you conquer your goal of achieving long-term health through stable glucose levels. Now that we've talked about glucose, let's move on to the next key to solving chronic health problems - stimulation.

KEY 3 – STIMULATION

THE ROLE OF STIMULATION

The definition of neurostimulation is "the activation of a nerve through an external source." Touch, for example, is a kind of stimulation as well as walking, cycling or swimming. Seeing something new is a form of stimulation. Hearing your friend speak is a form of stimulation. Picking up a 5lb weight and doing a bicep curl is a type of stimulation. When it comes to the neurological system, neural pathways need stimulation in order to be healthy. These pathways are designed to send information and signals (both electrically and chemically) from the body to the brain and the brain to the body, and don't forget your organ system is part of your body. Think of the neurological system like a muscle. If it's stimulated, it grows and gets stronger. If it's not stimulated, it begins to atrophy just like a muscle that isn't used enough.

It's crucial to understand the role that stimulation plays in solving chronic health problems because this is an area of health that's so often overlooked. Stimulation is required to stabilize neurological function. When a system is under-stimulated, it begins to atrophy and so does the area of the brain that controls that body part. To solve this problem, I use targeted, specific types of stimulation to "fire" those pathways. This activation creates more neuro-plasticity and increases the function of that area of the neurological systems. Neuro-plasticity (also known as "brain plasticity") is the ability of the brain and nervous system to modify its connections or rewire itself. Stimulating certain areas of the nervous system in specific ways makes the brain fire better which can solve problems in the body.

Different parts of the body are connected to different parts of the brain. For instance, if you are having problems with smell, taste, memory, or vision, all of those senses fire through your temporal lobe which means that part of your brain needs a certain kind of stimulation to get it working again. The reason we have to understand stimulation is because we need to find out what part of the brain is malfunctioning and figure out which systems we need to stimulate to bring that part of the brain back online.

For example, if a patient breaks their arm, their arm is going to atrophy within two weeks. They can eat broccoli and cauliflower and asparagus every day, five times per day, but if they don't stimulate the arm muscles, they're going to get smaller. The only way to make this muscle grow is to stimulate it. Specifically, a person with a broken arm, once the arm is out of the cast, needs the stimulation of bicep curls and tricep extensions to bring it and the part of their brain that controls their arm back to full working capacity. Doing calf raises, even though it's a form of stimulation, wouldn't help heal their arm because it's the wrong kind of stimulation. This method is known as "receptor-based activation," and it uses movement and stimulation to activate the brain.

Certain parts of the brain perform certain functions and control specific parts of the body. When we experience problems in our body, it's often because certain parts of the brain are not functioning as they should. Stimulating different parts of the brain in specific ways makes it "fire" or signal better which in turn solves problems in the body, and some of the stories that have come from treating patients through receptor-based activation have been nothing short of amazing.

A few years ago, a man came into the clinic and was having a major shoulder problem. In fact, his shoulder movement was so poor that he could barely get his arms to the level of his shoulders. He'd been to five different doctors and undergone many different forms of treatment, yet nothing had helped him move his arms normally. After I talked with him and did a neurological examination, it became clear that he needed receptor-based activation in his flexion / extension muscle groups. We worked together for about 30 and immediately afterwards, he was able to move his arms all the way over his head without any assistance. Why did this treatment work so fast? Because stimulating the correct area of the brain helped it become balanced, and it functioned more optimally because of it. Correct neurological stimulation is an amazing modality.

RESULTS OF STIMULATION

What actually happens when the body has a deficiency of stimulation? To understand the inner workings of the human brain, we first need to wrap our minds around the massive amount of energy that it requires to operate. The brain weighs about three pounds, and it is very metabolically demanding, consuming 25-30% of our overall oxygen and glucose intake. Consider that for a moment. Almost one third of the oxygen and glucose brought into our bodies is used by the brain alone. It is by far the most energy demanding organ, and because of that, the brain requires a constant supply of oxygen and glucose.

If the brain has the right amounts of oxygen and glucose, the final key that it needs to maintain optimal health is - you guessed it - proper neurological stimulation. It's the final piece of the Big Three (oxygen, glucose, stimulation) for maintaining a healthy, vibrant neurological system. If there's a lack of stimulation, the neurons will begin to break down and no longer produce the electrical and chemical activation to maintain neuronal health, which in turn causes the neurological pathways to atrophy. The atrophy of the pathways also causes atrophy in the brain. If you don't use it you lose it. In order for the neurological system to be healthy, it must be stimulated. If you want your arms to be strong, you have to do push-ups. If you don't, you'll have skinny, weak arms. If you don't stimulate your brain and neurological pathways, they break down as well, and the first signs of loss of brain health is brain fog, and the loss of focus, attention and concentration.

If the idea of your brain atrophying and your neurological pathways malfunctioning doesn't sound pleasant, I have good news for you. There may be a solution to your problem! You can increase the level of neurological stimulation and improve your health in a multitude of ways. When you increase stimulation in your daily life, you may experience an increased memory capacity, better vision, a clearer memory, a better sense of taste and smell, and more appreciation for touch. With all of these exciting benefits to gain, let's dig into strategies for self-testing and improving stimulation in your daily life.

YOUR FIRST STEPS – EVALUATION AND STIMULATION

There are several simple ways to test the health of your neurological pathways. The first indicator of a healthy brain is your ability to learn new information, to stay focused, and to concentrate on the topic at hand. When is the last time you learned something for the first time? The only long-term way to maintain the health of your brain is to stimulate it by trying new things, tasting new foods, smelling new smells, seeing new sights, and going to new places. Pay attention to how mentally "rigid" you are towards new ideas or plans. People who are inflexible and have a "my way or the highway" mentality often have very unhealthy brains.

When I examine the health of a patient's brain, there are four main areas of the brain that I consider: the temporal lobe, the parietal lobe, the frontal lobe, and the prefrontal lobe (or prefrontal cortex). The temporal lobe controls taste, smell, memory, and vision. The parietal lobe is in charge of body sensation and vision. The frontal lobe controls voluntary movement, and the prefrontal cortex handles focus, attention, concentration, memory, impulse control, and motivation. The deficiency of stimulation also determines which part of the brain is malfunctioning, and this is all determined through neurological testing. I have many tests that I do at my clinic, but there are also easy, at-home testing strategies for each lobe of the brain.

Temporal lobe self-test: Ask yourself these questions: "Can I taste and smell things as I did before? Have my senses increased, decreased or stayed the same? (If they've decreased, that indicates a lack of stimulation in the temporal lobe). How's my memory? Am I as "sharp" as ever or has my memory declined?"

Parietal lobe self-test: One simple test is called the Digit Span Test. Here's how you perform it. You need a partner. Close your eyes and have your partner touch two of your toes on one foot. Can you identify how many toes are between the toes your partner is touching? Now repeat on the other foot as well as your fingers on both hands. If this neurological system is damaged, you will not be able to identify what your partner is doing.

Frontal lobe self-test: Do I move as well now as I did in the past or has my movement slowed? How is my memory compared to years past? Am I becoming more irritated over trivial things? Am I becoming more inflexible? The biggest problem with frontal lobe issues is that you don't see the change but everyone around you does. It's strange but with frontal lobe demise, we can't see it in ourselves but everyone else can see our deficiencies.

Prefrontal cortex self-test: A healthy prefrontal cortex is essential for planning, and execution of complex issues such as behavior, speech, and logical reasoning, as well as impulse control, motivation, understanding the consequences of your actions, and short term memory. If you've noticed you're not following through with what you've started, planning poorly, having short term memory as well as lacking impulse control, then your prefrontal cortex may need some rehab.

CEREBELLUM:

Stability test (do this with caution): Put your feet together (side-by-side), close your eyes, and hold that position for 15 seconds. Next, put your right foot in front of the left, close your eyes and hold for 15 seconds. Lastly, put your left foot in front of your right foot, close your eyes, and hold for 15 seconds.

Flex test (do this with caution): Stand on one leg with the other leg lifted and flexed at 90 degrees, then hold that position for 15 seconds. Repeat on the other side.

These cerebellar tests are very important for stability and balance. Count out loud and see how long you can maintain your balance and stability. A healthy cerebellum will allow for the full fifteen seconds for each test.

These simple at-home tests can give you an idea of how your neurological pathways are currently firing, and if you performed the tests and didn't like the results, don't fear. Here are some exercises you can do to stimulate those pathways and "fire" your brain back up.

Non-linear complex movements: You can actually do these exercises while you're sitting down at the table or relaxing on your couch. Start by sitting down or standing up, then do a figure eight in the air with your arm or "write" the name of your city and state in the air, write your ABCs, your name, etc. Try writing your name in the air with your hand and leg at the same time. This fires your cerebellum, frontal lobe and the parietal lobe at that same time. Pair this with deep breathing and you're really stimulating your brain and giving it plenty of oxygen to increase the level of stimulation your neurological system can take.

Deep breathing exercises: As stated before deep breathing or forced breathing stimulates frontal lobe function. Start slowly and build up and remember the 1:2 ratio. Breathe in four seconds and out eight seconds. Once you can perform 4:8 move up to 6:12, six seconds in and twelve seconds out. Next step is 8:16, eight seconds in and sixteen seconds out. It won't be easy getting to 8:16 but remember, things worth having are hardly ever easy.

CHAPTER 8

KEY 4 – AUTOIMMUNE DISORDERS

THE ROLE OF AUTOIMMUNE (AI) DISORDERS

Before we dig into autoimmune disorders and their profound impact on your health, let's first look at the driver of autoimmunity which is your immune system. So what is an immune system, exactly, and why is it important to your body? Your immune system is basically your built-in SEAL Team 6. It's your body's special defense mechanism against all of the antigens of the world. An antigen is any substance that sparks your immune system to produce antibodies such as chemicals, bacteria, cancer cells, viruses, or pollen. Your immune system recognizes that these antigens are not meant to be inside of you and then activates to fight off and kill the offender. When you develop an autoimmune condition, your immune system begins attacking your own tissues because it thinks your tissue is the antigen. Essentially, an autoimmune condition is "friendly fire" within your body.

Autoimmune (AI) conditions can be devastating to patients suffering with chronic health problems because AI can not only exacerbate existing chronic problems, but AI by itself is the health problem. The autoimmune condition acts like the Tasmanian devil inside your body, wreaking havoc and causing damage. Once an autoimmune condition begins destroying things, it can cause a whole host of other seemingly unrelated issues.

One of the biggest drivers of autoimmune conditions that I see in my clinic is a sensitivity to gluten. Gluten is a protein found in wheat and is in manufactured cereal, grains, pasta, bread and flour, just to name a few products. It is the substance that makes bread dough elastic and stretchy, and it is devastating to the human brain. Gluten is one of the most destructive proteins found on the planet today, and no, it's not the same wheat that our ancestors consumed centuries ago. It's a commercialized, hybridized version that our body can no longer recognize or break down. As a result, undigested gluten proteins work their way into the bloodstream and spark an immune response. Since gluten's amino acid profile closely resembles the amino acid profile of the human thyroid gland and cerebellum tissue, this immune response quickly turns into an autoimmune response that attacks those parts of your body.

Every single human needs to test their tolerance for gluten, and the test I recommend is panel A2 from www.Enterolab. com. You can order this test directly from the company. Another test is Cyrex Array 3, but a doctor has to order this test. This is a genetic test which identifies whether or not you carry the gluten sensitivity gene and if it has been turned on. It also tells you whether or not you have the Celiac gene. I can't stress enough how important it is for everyone to become educated on gluten intolerance and their body's reaction to wheat and other cereal grains.

RESULTS FROM AUTOIMMUNE DISORDERS

When your body is battling an autoimmune disorder, it could appear as a multitude of other, seemingly unrelated chronic health problems. Ataxia, which is an unstable posture or irregular gait, is commonly linked to autoimmune disease. Thyroid problems like Hashimoto's Disease can be rooted in autoimmune conditions. Recent research has suggested approximately 90% of people who have thyroid issues also have an autoimmune disorder. Fibromyalgia is a chronic disorder characterized by widespread musculoskeletal pain, fatigue, and tenderness in localized areas and is often rooted in autoimmune problems. Cerebellum issues like blurred vision, balance problems, and uncoordinated movements with your hands and feet are all signals that you may be dealing with an autoimmune condition.

Other signs of autoimmune disease are general cognitive decline like a lack of focus, attention and concentration. Dementia, forgetting things like names, numbers, and dates, is a concerning signal of an autoimmune condition. Psychological disorders like panic, anxiety, depression, and irrational fear are often rooted in autoimmune causes as well. Migraine headaches, multiple sclerosis, ALS (often called Lou Gehrig's disease), stiffness in movements, tremors, and restless leg syndrome are all chronic conditions that are closely linked to autoimmune roots with the majority of these reactions being triggered by the gluten found in modern wheat.

Many people mistakenly think that only people diagnosed with Celiac disease are intolerant to gluten, however the truth is that only about 30% of people who have Celiac disease have gut-related issues. The other 70% have a myriad of other problems.

Celiac disease destroys the microvilli, the tiny hair-like projections within the small intestine that increase nutrient absorption. These projections increase the surface area of the small intestine allowing more area for nutrients to be absorbed. Celiac destroys these microvilli to the point that they can't absorb nutrients. When they are damaged, it kicks off a host of other disease processes that can turn into full-blown autoimmune conditions.

YOUR FIRST STEP

When the gut becomes inflamed and damaged, harmful proteins like gluten cross the blood-brain barrier and "dock" in the part of your brain where your opioid receptors live. This means people who regularly eat breads, cakes, cookies, brownies, and other foods containing wheat flour are truly addicted to these foods. When they eat them, their brain reacts very similarly to someone consuming opioids. What's your reaction as you've read my encouragement to ditch wheat and gluten? Did you say, "No way! I can't live without my (fill in the blank)." If those thoughts crossed your mind, there's a good chance you're addicted to gluten.

I can't encourage you strongly enough - get gluten out of your life. The side effects are absolutely devastating. If you want to learn more about the bad effects of gluten, I highly recommend the book *Grain Brain* by David Perlmutter, MD. It goes into much more detail on the effects that modern gluten has on the human brain.

If you suspect that you have a lurking autoimmune condition, don't lose hope. It may be possible to slow down the damage, and in some cases even reverse it IF caught early enough. Here comes "tough love part two." The most important point for you to remember is this: improving the lives of patients suffering with chronic health problems begins with my patients taking personal responsibility. Most autoimmune conditions are triggered by lifestyle choices which means that they can also be improved upon through major lifestyle changes. These kinds of changes can be challenging to make, but what is your health worth to you? That's the question you need to answer when you look in the mirror, "Am I worth it?' Only you can answer that question.

The first step to identifying an autoimmune condition is to order the www.EnteroLab.com panel A2 test. If I was a betting kind of guy, I would wager that you do have the gluten sensitivity gene. If you have a gluten sensitivity problem, it's crucial that you avoid gluten at all costs and get on an autoimmune paleo diet. You also need to start the Brain-Body-Gut 90 detox.

Will you make mistakes? Absolutely! Anyone taking on a major lifestyle change will slip up and fall off "the bandwagon" as we say, but don't let those mistakes keep you from getting back on the program. Keep heading in the right direction and you will begin to see improvement.

A great first step in the right direction is to deep clean your home of all products containing gluten. This includes cooking devices like toasters that have touched your bread, English muffins, etc. Throw away all wheat flours, breads, cookies, baking mixes, and more. With a wheat and gluten sensitivity, you're either all in or you're out. You can't be 95% in, you have to be 100% committed because once you consume gluten, it takes months for it to completely leave your system.

Take heart. There is hope. You can get rid of all the negative side effects of gluten while still enjoying your life. However, it takes time and commitment for these changes to become part of your new lifestyle. If you're willing to put in the work, I can almost guarantee you'll see a significant improvement in your health. Now that we've covered autoimmune disorders, let's move to the next key to solving chronic health problems.

CHAPTER 9

KEY 5 – INFLAMMATION

THE ROLE OF INFLAMMATION

Inflammation - this is a term we hear often, but do we really know what it is, why it happens, and why we often have too much of it? Let's start by discussing what inflammation is supposed to do. In its proper context, inflammation is actually a good thing because it acts as a signaling agent to tell the body to start repairing, restoring, and regenerating itself. This regeneration is kicked off by the formation of new blood vessels. Nothing can heal until new blood vessels are created (called angiogenesis), and in this regard, inflammation is a positive thing.

Inflammation comes to the rescue when you experience an acute injury like a twisted ankle, a dislocated shoulder, or a badly banged shin. In that context, inflammation is a localized physical condition that causes the body to become swollen, red, and hot to the touch. This is when inflammation signals to the rest of the body to begin the healing process. The trouble begins when inflammation gets out of hand and out of homeostasis.

Homeostasis is the body's ability to maintain a relatively stable internal state that persists despite changes in the world outside. When there isn't homeostasis, disease processes can begin to develop. As with many parts of our health, inflammation causes problems when it goes rogue and there is too much of it.

Inflammation becomes a major issue when it's continually present in the body. This can happen for a variety of reasons. In this scenario, inflammation in the body is like fire inside of a house. It's totally destructive and stands in the way of optimizing chronic issues. Some of the most common signs of chronic inflammation are actually more psychological than physical. Brain fog, depression, anxiety, irritability, and fatigue are all signs of chronic inflammation of the brain. When chronic inflammation exists in the brain, that dreaded brain fog is almost always the first symptom to appear. Sometimes I compare it to feeling like the "walking dead" or like you're living in zombie land. You have a hard time focusing, concentrating, and staying hooked on one task for an extended period of time.

Inflammation plays a distinct and important role in healing chronic disease because it's something we must eliminate before we can begin untangling the web of dysfunction and healing the root issue. If a house was on fire, would you start rebuilding it before the fire was completely put out? No, that would be ridiculous. In the same way, we have to eradicate the chronic inflammation before we can begin rebuilding the body. If there's chronic inflammation present, it's going to accelerate the degeneration in your brain, joints, nervous system, and circulatory system much more quickly. If you're dealing with any kind of inflammation anywhere, you have to zap it before you can start to heal.

Bloodwork is the most accurate way to measure the level of inflammation present in the body. The A1C markers on a blood panel can be used to measure inflammation. The CRP (c-reactive protein) and the homocysteine markers also indicate inflammation levels. Everyone has some level of inflammation present in their system at all times, but these tests are used to see if it is out of control or not. This information is used to make a plan for reducing the level of chronic inflammation in your system.

RESULTS OF INFLAMMATION

So what causes this kind of chronic inflammation? The factors can be both psychological and physical. Psychological things like being overworked, excessively difficult workouts, unhealthy relationships, a stressful job, and not having enough "me time" can all contribute to chronic inflammation of the brain.

Physical causes of chronic inflammation can be obvious things like slipping and falling, a car wreck (even if it was several years ago), whiplash, repetitive injuries or motions, falling out of a tree, falling off a ladder, and more. Chronic inflammation from these kinds of traumatic injuries can stay with you many years, even after the more obvious symptoms disappear.

A glucose imbalance (see Chapter 6), anemia, leaky gut syndrome, leaky brain syndrome, and food sensitivities can cause out-of-control inflammation in the body. When these things occur, the body releases cortisol to combat the stress of the inflammatory process. Cortisol is a stress-related hormone that is meant to help control blood sugar levels, regulate metabolism, help reduce inflammation, and assist with memory formulation. However, when the body signals cortisol to be released over and over again, the negative effects begin to spiral out of control. If there's too much cortisol in your system, it can affect the quality of your sleep. It also directly attacks the hippocampus, the region of the brain that is associated primarily with memory.

Decreasing the level of inflammation in your system will positively affect your health in many, many ways. First of all, it will save your brain. That sounds extreme, but it's true. The brain is very sensitive to inflammation, and by decreasing the level of inflammation in the brain, you're going to avoid many memory, focus and concentration, and anxiety driven problems. When you put out the "fire in the house," your focus, attention, and brain fog should significantly decrease. You should have an increased ability to think more clearly and experience a clarity of mind and senses that you haven't noticed for quite a while. As you work to decrease the inflammation in your body, your pain syndromes should start to decrease. Your joint pain may slow down or be completely eliminated, and you may even notice your balance improving.

If your inflammation levels are out of control, the first thing to do is look at is your diet. You can take all the anti-inflammatory products in the world, but you can't out-supplement a poor diet. You can't out-medicate it either. Making the necessary dietary changes (most commonly, eliminating gluten, sugar, and casein, the protein found in milk) is a major first step to reducing inflammation and healing chronic disease.

YOUR FIRST STEPS

So what can you do, starting today, to begin decreasing the inflammation level in your body? What a great question! The exciting thing is that there is a lot you can do to help put out the fire and set the stage for true healing. First let's talk about psychological and physiological things you can do to reduce one of the biggest drivers of inflammation, which is stress.

If you notice stress playing a major inflammatory role in your life, start incorporating important mental health practices like regular deep tissue massage and "unplugging" from technology on a regular basis. No one is going to care more about your brain and bodily health than you, and you need to make these things a major priority in your life. All of these things are an investment in your long-term health. Make a commitment to disconnect from technology for one day per week. Schedule a ninety minute massage once per month. Listen to soothing music. Go to a happy, funny movie and laugh for a whole hour straight. Listen to soothing nature sounds. Eliminate the bad and unnecessarily stressful relationships from your life. If you're in a bad relationship, discontinue it or take the hard but necessary steps to improve it. All of these small changes add up to a major effect. It's like a snowball that's rolling down a hill. At first, the changes seem minor, but as you pick up speed, the momentum becomes undeniable.

As far as physical changes that can help decrease inflammation, there are a lot of them. First of all, stop eating gluten, casein, and sugar. These substances do nothing but cause inflammation and wreak havoc on your gut-brain health. Stop eating processed foods that are filled with inflammatory oils and Trans Fats. Examples of trans fats include, but are not limited to, store bought cakes, cookies and pies, shortening, microwave popcorn, frozen pizza, fried foods, doughnuts, non-dairy creamer, and margarine. No wonder you're having headaches, brain fog and your feet are tingling and numb. In addition to dietary changes, you can incorporate other physical things like using an inversion table or adding nutritional supplements into your daily routine.

I think everyone should be taking an omega-3 fish oil supplement, and lots of it. The bare minimum daily required amount is 500mg but you can take up to 5000mg with zero negative side effects. Take the best kind you can afford. If you've had a bad experience with Omega-3 supplements in the past, it may be because you took a poor quality supplement. Up your intake of foods high in antioxidants, aka super foods. This includes things like purple, red or blue grapes (make sure they have seeds in them and eat the seeds as well), blueberries, raspberries, raw almonds, walnuts, pecans, kale, spinach (see, Popeye was right), broccoli, sweet potatoes, green or black tea, beans, and fish. These substances help rid the body of free radicals caused by inflammation. Drink real, home-brewed green tea. I recommend buying through Tea Market Spice in Seattle, Washington (phone number 800-735-7198.) My favorite varieties are the Japanese green tea (#3577) and the China mountain green tea (#5577).

When you begin to incorporate these lifestyle changes into your daily routine, you will be amazed at the way your body and brain feel. Eliminating inflammation in your body is a fantastic step toward healing chronic health problems and regaining your health and vibrancy. Now that we've talked about inflammation, let's move onto the next key - environmental toxins.

CHAPTER 10

KEY 6 – NEUROTOXINS

THE ROLE OF NEUROTOXINS

A neurotoxin is something you ingest into your body that has a direct link to brain and neurological destruction. The word "neurotoxin" may spark images of strange green substances bubbling in chemistry class, but the reality is that neurotoxins are hiding in some of the most ingested substances on earth. In fact, you probably have many of these substances in your kitchen right now, and understanding the role these toxins play in either starting or continuing chronic health problems is crucial. As your body digests and breaks down a neurotoxic substance, it may either trigger an autoimmune attack or kick off some kind of destructive brain and/or body disease process.

Here's a list of the most common neurotoxins that the majority of Americans consume every day:

- Wheat, particularly the gluten (the protein found in wheat), is the most destructive protein you can ever put in your body therefore it is classified as a neurotoxin. Again, I recommend the book *Grain Brain* by David Perlmutter, MD.

- Common table sugar is also a neurotoxin. As your body breaks it down, your blood sugar becomes spiked, which triggers a release of insulin which in turn produces a destructive inflammatory response.

- High fructose corn syrup is highly inflammatory. Most commonly used as a sweetener in sodas and other sweet drinks, high fructose corn syrup triggers a similar inflammatory response as table sugar. Because of this, I highly suggest you stop drinking sodas immediately.

- Artificial sweeteners are very toxic to the brain. Though they seem innocent because they don't contain sugar, they harm the brain in a different way. They contain a substance that causes our bodies' glutamate, an excitatory neurotransmitter, to over react to the product. It's similar to slamming the gas pedal of your car to the floor while it's in park and over-revving the engine to the point of blowing it up. These artificial sweeteners do the same thing to your glutamate neurotransmitters and essentially blow their doors off. To avoid artificial sweeteners, stop drinking diet soda as well as other diet beverages. For more information on the topic, I recommend you read *Excitotoxins: The Taste That Kills* by Russell Blaylock, MD.

- Monosodium Glutamate (MSG) is another substance that has a similar effect on your sensory neurotransmitters as the artificial sweeteners. This substance over-excites those receptors to the point of malfunction and degeneration which then leads to negative psychological side effects like brain fog, depression, and anxiety. To avoid MSG, steer clear of processed foods like flavored tortilla chips, ranch dressing mixes, some soy sauces and prepackaged Asian foods, and other highly processed items.

- Trans fats are hydrogenated oils that are highly inflammatory to the body. Anything that is inflammatory over a long period of time is going to destroy your brain function so avoiding anything that contains trans fats is crucial.

- Drinking bottled water from the commonly sold plastic disposable bottles has proven to be a source of neurotoxic material. Avoiding the consumption of and exposure to these plastic products greatly reduces the toxic load on your body's detoxification systems.

- There are a few more common neurotoxic culprits like heavy metals - lead, mercury, and formaldehyde, and these toxic substances are found in some unsuspecting places. Recent medical studies have shown that lead poisoning may be generational. The results showed that if a parent got lead poisoning, it took roughly 4 generations to get it out of their offspring's system. Mercury (aka thermasol) is found in vaccines, as well as aluminum, which is in most underarm deodorants.

RESULTS FROM NEUROTOXINS

Understanding the realities and effects of neurotoxins plays an important role in helping people optimize their chronic issues. Since these neurotoxins damage the brain, the body's most important healing organ, it only stands to reason that removing substances which hurt the brain will accelerate healing. When there's a large amount of neurotoxins present in your body, it accelerates the degeneration of your joints, causes focus and concentration issues, can increase fear and anxiety, activate autoimmune disorders and destroy body tissue. Many chronic diseases, movement disorders, fibromyalgia, burning and numbness, tingling and coordination problems can be linked to an overload of neurotoxins.

These negative effects are often overlooked because most people, even traditional doctors, don't understand the link between inflammation of the brain and one's ability to improve their chronic condition. A brain and body detox as well as an elimination diet are very useful tools for changing your body's chemistry and your lifestyle so you can kick these nasty toxins to the curb.

Decreasing your consumption of neurotoxins will also yield some very nice lifestyle benefits like better sleep (the more cortisol you have, the less melatonin you release therefore making it harder to fall asleep and stay asleep), decreased pain and discomfort, better bowel movements, improved sexual function, better concentration and focus, and greater stability and balance.

YOUR FIRST STEPS

Your first step is to remember that you have the power to stop eating, drinking, and surrounding yourself with foods and substances that are neurotoxic to your brain. Stop eating the processed foods and quit drinking sodas, both traditional and diet. Stop buying plastic water bottles and instead invest in a glass water bottle that you refill at home with reverse osmosis water. If you have coffee, make sure you drink only organic coffee. Flavor your water with lemon or lime juice instead of ingesting traditional soda drinks or artificial sweeteners. There are many, many ways to enjoy the things you love like a great cup of coffee or a refreshing beverage without sacrificing your health.

The bottom line is to eliminate the neurotoxins listed above. Are there other toxins out there besides the ones I talked about in this book? Absolutely. There are herbicides, pesticides, environmental toxins, and more, but your exposure to those are mostly out of your control. Instead of focusing on what we can't control, let's focus on what we can control. You get to control everything you put in your mouth and on your body. Those daily choices are either healing you or slowly killing you, and you get to decide which direction you choose.

CHAPTER 11

KEY 7 — THE BRAIN-GUT CONNECTION

THE ROLE OF GUT HEALTH

What is your "gut?" What does it have to do with healing chronic disease and untangling the web of dysfunction? Why does the condition of your gut matter so much for your overall health picture? How is gut health connected to the well-being of your brain? We're going to answer all of these important questions and more in this chapter.

For starters, your "gut" is not referring to the roundness we get around our midsection when we eat too many Christmas cookies. Instead, the term "gut health" refers to the physical state and physiologic function of the many parts of the gastrointestinal tract, also called the Enteric Nervous System. At one time, our digestive system was considered a relatively "simple" body system, but as our understanding of the gut and its many functions has grown, it's proven to be anything but simple. The gut not only consists of many different organs which work together to withdraw nutrition from our food, it also is home to trillions of microorganisms which live in our intestines. These microorganisms are a mixture of beneficial and non-beneficial bacteria, and in a healthy, optimally functioning gut, the "good bugs" far outnumber the "bad bugs." What's even more amazing is that these microorganisms are an essential part of your immune system, and over 70% of your immune system is found in your gut. The health and wellness of these microorganisms greatly depends on the foods we eat, the stress we endure, the medications we take, and the environment we live in.

In recent years, more attention has been paid to the importance of gut health and the way an unhealthy gut contributes to the web of dysfunction. The gut is so crucial to our overall wellness for more reasons than digesting food and extracting nutrients. Your gut (Enteric Nervous System) is connected to your brain via the Vagus Nerve, and in fact, they're so connected that we should almost view them as one system. If one is damaged, dysfunction in the other is sure to follow.

The link between the gut and the brain is known as the "gut/brain axis." The two are so interconnected that they're basically one, ultra complex system. The human gut (Enteric Nervous System) is lined with more than 500 million nerve cells so it's practically a brain unto itself. To give you an example, the human spinal cord has approximately 100 million nerve cells. Because the Gut/Brain axis is so interconnected, in order to heal one, you have to also heal the other. The neuro-metabolic web of dysfunction really starts to untangle when you solve the problems with your Gut/Brain Axis.

There are two main ways that the brain and the gut communicate with one another, and either of these modes of communication can be disrupted by trauma or inflammation. The first way the brain and gut communicate is through the Vagus nerve, a large "super highway" kind of nerve that extends from the brain stem to part of the colon. It also happens to be the longest cranial nerve in the body.

The second way the gut and the brain communicate is through the Central Autonomic Network which is also known as the

"C.A.N." This complex network can be compromised by trauma as well as physiological or psychological issues. Any kind of damage to either the function of the Vagus nerve or the C.A.N. may spark leaky gut syndrome in your body. In fact, research suggests that within 6-12 hours after trauma happens to the brain (concussion, whiplash injury), you will have a leaky gut.

Your digestive system plays a key role in protecting your body from harmful substances. The walls of the intestines act as barriers, kind of like screen doors in our home, controlling what enters the bloodstream to be transported to your organs. If that screen is compromised, the barrier is breached and bugs get into the house. We have these kinds of protective barriers in our brain and gut and when they're damaged, trouble occurs. The inflammatory cascade starts here.

Small gaps in the intestinal wall called "tight junctions" allow water and nutrients to pass through, while blocking the passage of harmful substances. When these tight junctions are damaged to the point that they open up and no longer prevent harmful substances from passing into the bloodstream, it is known as "leaky gut syndrome." Leaky gut can be summarized in two words – intestinal permeability. When the gut is "leaky" and bacteria and other antigens enter the bloodstream, it can cause widespread inflammation and potentially trigger a reaction from the immune system. Those harmful substances are supposed to simply pass through the digestive tract, and when they breach that barrier and get into your bloodstream, they wreak all kinds of havoc.

Gluten sensitivity as well as an overload of neurotoxins can also cause damage and result in a leaky gut. The reason that gut health is so crucial is because if your gut isn't healthy and doing its job, it affects every other system in the body. To solve the riddle of chronic health issues and begin to untangle the neuro-metabolic web of dysfunction, we have to address brain function and gut function. That's why gut health is one of my seven keys to healing chronic health issues.

Gut health plays a distinct role in fostering true health and healing chronic disease because of the key role it plays in your immune system. As I mentioned earlier, about 70% of your immune system is found in your gut. To foster true health, you also need homeostasis between your sympathetic and parasympathetic nervous systems. Your Vagus nerve, the nerve that runs from the brainstem all the way to the colon, is what controls all of these functions.

To measure your gut health, there are several good blood work tests that show whether your gut is functioning correctly or not. The www.EnteroLab.com panel A2 test indicates if the gut is functioning properly. If you have an immune response to milk, wheat, soy or eggs, you likely have a leaky gut. If you have a leaky gut, you have a leaky brain.

RESULTS FROM GUT HEALTH

When you have poor gut health, there are a whole host of problems that could be showing up in your life. Some of the physical maladies you may be experiencing include GERD (gastroesophageal reflux disease), Crohn's disease, irritable bowel syndrome, SIBO (small intestinal bacterial overgrowth), and gastric reflux. These common disease processes all find their roots in having a leaky gut.

Many psychological issues like brain fog, lack of focus and attention, depression, anxiety, and overwhelming fear can develop as a result of leaky gut because when the gut is not healthy, neither is the brain. As I said before, you cannot have a healthy brain unless you have a healthy gut. If you have damage to the brain or you're feeding your gut bad stuff, those barriers are compromised and it kicks off a wave of inflammation and autoimmune disorders.

YOUR FIRST STEPS

So what can you do, starting today, to increase your gut health?

1. Eliminate the seven most common neurotoxins (see chapter 10). If you damage your brain, you damage your gut and vice versa.

2. Complete the Brain-Body-Gut 90 day detox program. Detoxifying your body and supporting your gut and brain health will kick start your path to healing and help you begin to untangle the web of dysfunction.

3. Do the nerve stimulation exercises below 3-4 times per week. Since the Vagus nerve is the main super highway which allows the gut and brain to communicate, stimulating the Vagus nerve regularly is a fantastic way to promote optimal gut health.

I also suggest some extremely high quality nutritional supplements. The supplements listed below are NOT FDA approved to treat and disease or cure any aliment, and is NOT to take the place of any medication your doctor may have prescribed.

i. *Apex Energetics – ClearVite-PSF (K-84) Part 1 of 3 of our Brain-Body-Gut 90 day detox. Helps support liver detoxification reactions, the biliary system, and sugar metabolism.*

ii. *Apex Energetics – RepairVite (K-60) Part 2 of 3 of our Brain-Body-Gut 90 day detox program. Intended to support the intestinal tract and intestinal lining.*

iii. *Apex Energetics – Strengtia Probiotics (K-61) Part 3 of 3 of our Brain-Body-Gut 90 day detox program. Designed to fortify the intestinal microbial environment with targeted probiotics.*

iv. *Apex Energetics – Omega-CO3 (K-7) intended to support the brain and the immune system.*

v. *Apex Energetics – Protoglysen (K-28) and Glysen (K-1) Both are designed to support sugar metabolism and help buffer glycemic response.*

vi. *Apex Energetics - NeurO2 (K-45) uniquely designed and mechanistically balanced to support the cerebral microvascular for healthy blood flow to the brain.*

vii. *Apex Energetics – Neuro-Flam (K-46) is a phenol-flavonoid complex designed to specifically target brain health as it relates to microglial activity in the brain-immune system.*

viii. *Apex Energetics - Metacrin-DX (K-10) is a formula designed to support phase 1 and phase 2 detoxication.*

ix. *Apex Energetics – GlutenFlam (k-52) is a one-of-a-kind digestive aid that features powerful digestive enzymes to address unintended gluten and casein exposure.*

x. *Bionan-X Medical – Nano Amplified Hemp Extract Transdermal Cream*

xi. *Bionan-X Medical – Nano Amplified Hemp Extract Supplement Drops*

Keep in mind that if you drop a pebble in the water, the greatest impact is the ripple directly next to the surface of the water where the pebble made contact. The same is true with stimulating neural pathways. However, there's always a ripple effect which flows out to benefit more systems in the body that you may be initially trying to help. When you think about stimulating the neural pathways, the more that you can fire at a time, the greater the positive effects that come from that stimulation. The following exercises will help you "fire" the Vagus nerve and keep it active and healthy.

4. At-home Vagus Nerve Stimulation Exercises

Gargling: Gargle for two minutes straight, and I mean gargle like your life depends on it. To accentuate the effect of this stimulation, try fixating on a certain point or part of the wall that's above you. To multiply the positive effects of this even more, do these two things while also doing non-linear complex movements like writing out your name in "air letters" with your free hand or spelling your first and last name.

Ear Lobes: Massaging your outer ear lobes stimulates the Vagus nerve.

The "No No" Exercise: As you focus your attention on a point on the wall, put your feet together and fixate on that point while also rotating your head from right to left *and* humming the "Happy Birthday" song. Then change the exercise by moving your head back and forth as if you're saying "yes yes."

Humming: Humming seems to activate very beneficial parts of the brain that are connected to the Vagus nerve and therefore essential to your gut health.

Gagging: If you're brave enough, try gagging yourself approximately three times until you tear up. Sound intense? It is, but it's one of the best ways to stimulate the Vagus nerve.

If you start to implement these changes, you may begin to notice decreased bloating, gas and diarrhea. You'll notice less brain fog and enjoy improved gut function. We need to see our gut and brain as one because they directly communicate with one another. Now that we've covered your gut, let's move to the next key to solving chronic health problems.

PART THREE

SHARED FOLLOW THROUGH

CHAPTER 12

HOW EXAMS HELP YOU HEAL

WHAT IS AN EXAM?

In our clinic, every patient's journey begins with a thorough functional neurological exam. This is a head-to-toe neurological evaluation on you. We do this because we treat every single person as a unique, one-of-a-kind case. Think of the way a detective picks up the trail of a murder case that's gone cold. That's how we approach each person's tangled web of dysfunction. The exam is like cracking open that file and looking at every piece of evidence in a new light.

Many times, exams are used more as a "check off" list for doctors. They're such a rich opportunity for the doctor to gather valuable data about their patient, yet they don't bother to ask enough questions or get the right kind of data needed to really solve the patient's problems. Too often, doctors come in with preconceived notions and they don't put their hands on their patients. Yes, you actually have to touch your patient to do a neurological exam.

In my experience, performing a thorough neurological exam is both an art and a science. The art aspect focuses on how to perform the exam fluidly and in a systematic way that identifies which systems are not functioning properly and are likely damaged. It's also an art form to identify and then assist the most devastated areas of the patient's brain. The science portion comes from all the neurology in classroom learning at the universities as well as textbooks. Most doctors can do the science part. It's the art part that's rare.

I use the same acronym to guide me through every single patient exam, and it's called POPQRST.

P - Primary complaint. What health issue is having the biggest negative impact on their life? Has anyone else in their family had this issue before?

O - Onset. When did the symptoms start? And is the primary complaint staying the same or getting worse?

P - Pain. What provokes the pain and what makes it better?

Q - Quality of pain. Is there burning, numbness, or tingling?

R - Radiate. Does the pain radiate out or does it stay local?

S - Severity. Rank the pain on a scale of 1-10. How bad is it?

T - Time. What time of day or night is the primary complaint worse?

During this exam, we also test the patient's oxygen levels to determine if they're anemic or not. The body can't heal unless it has the proper supply of oxygen, so this is a crucial first step. We also take their blood pressure (which gives us another hint about their oxygen levels), draw blood and perform intensive blood work, and do glucose testing. All of these tests are getting baseline measurements on the patient's seven keys to health because these keys provide the clues I use to untangle their web of dysfunction and heal their chronic health problems.

During the neurological testing portion of the exam, I use a tuning fork to test the sensitivity of their nervous system. I take the tuning fork, place it on their sternum, and allow them to feel the vibration. That vibration represents a value of 10 and serves as our reference point. Then, I do the same thing but put the tuning fork against their big toe, their thumbs and their shoulders.

Next, I do a two-point discrimination test where I make sure the radial nerve (the nerve which controls sensation in the back of the arm and forearm) is intact and functioning. Then, I test the lower extremities using a two point discrimination test. I check the L-4 saphenous nerve (controls sensation to the inside of the lower leg) and L-5 superficial peroneal nerve (controls the outside of the lower leg). I follow that test with the digit span test where I evaluate the Median nerve which controls the thumb and first and second fingers. I then check Ulnar nerve sensation to part of the ring finger and little finger. Next, I perform the digit span test on the toes via the L-5 superficial peroneal nerve which controls all sensation on the top of the feet as well as all toes (except the small toe which is controlled by the S-1 sural nerve). These tests give me a good indication of how the patient's peripheral nervous system as well as the parietal lobe, located in the back half of the brain, is functioning. Next, I test their reflexes which tells me how well their motor reflexes are responding. Human beings have 10 motor reflexes, and I test all reflexes to see how well their cerebellum, brain and spinal cord are working.

CEREBELLUM TESTS:

After that, I ask them to stand up, if they can, and put their feet together and close their eyes. Next, I'll ask the patient to close their eyes and put their right foot in front of the left foot. Then, I have them switch legs. I follow that exercise up by asking them to alternately lift each leg off the ground and hold it at a 90 degree angle. If your cerebellum is functioning optimally you should be able to maintain each balance/stability test for fifteen seconds. I continue the neurological part of the exam by testing them for smell, fine motor skills, and many more factors that show me the state of their neurological health.

Finger to nose test: I ask the patient to close their eyes and try to place their little finger on the tip of their nose. Fingertip to nose tip. If they miss, they probably have a decreased functioning cerebellum on the side being tested.

It's important to approach an exam with humility and curiosity because I'm working in the field of probabilities, not absolutes. If you're aspiring to be an accountant or an engineer and seeking absolute answers, this probably is not the field for you. Practically nothing in neurology is absolute. Approaching the patient as if they're a completely new, one-of-a-kind case is the most important mental shift I make every time I prepare to do an exam.

THE FUNDAMENTALS OF AN EFFECTIVE EXAM

When a patient comes into the clinic for an exam, they'll have already filled out their paperwork and we have their blood work results on hand. I start the exam by asking them some questions. Then I move into the primary pillars of executing a great exam.

Pillar One: Where is the problem? Is it neurological, metabolic or both?

Pillar Two: How much can we stimulate the system before it fatigues?

Pillar Three: Do I think I can improve this patient's well being?

Often, the exam reveals new and insightful information that helps us "crack the case." One of my favorite stories is of a young lady who came into the clinic for an exam. She was twenty-one years old and had been a soccer player before her condition forced her to quit sports and drop out of school. She was afflicted with 15-20 seizures per day and had been to all of the major hospitals and experts in the country, yet she was still struggling. Any kind of major stimulation sent her into a seizing fit. If she got out of the car and the sun hit her eyes wrong, she started seizing.

Through neurological testing and the exam, I discovered she had a possible autoimmune disorder, and her oxygen levels were very low. Her feet and hands were also very cold which meant they weren't getting adequate oxygen. It turned out she had developed autoimmunity against her gut.

I prescribed a treatment plan of Vagal nerve stimulation, the 90 day brain and body detox, brain stimulation therapy, and many other home-based modalities. Once we identified the root cause of her problem, which was the autoimmune condition, we began this treatment protocol that targeted the root cause of her dysfunction. Within four months, she no longer had any seizures. Since then, she re-enrolled in school and wants to become a physical therapist. This is the power of doing the right kind of exam. The clues I found in the neurological exam helped me figure out what part of the body was malfunctioning, and when we addressed the root of the problem, she got her life back.

Another favorite story is of a patient who had been told he needed to move to an assisted living facility because of his poor health and lack of coordination. He initially came in for "frozen" shoulders that wouldn't move his arms above 90 degrees. Through a neurological exam, we discovered the part of the brain that was malfunctioning. We used brain stimulation therapy to activate certain muscle groups to reset the neurological receptors in that part of the body which allowed the brain to recognize and execute the full range of motion. Within four minutes of his first treatment, he went from being able to lift his arms from 90 degrees to lifting them above his head to 180 degrees. From that point, we worked together to heal a whole cascade of chronic health problems that were holding him back and limiting his quality of life. Within nine months of receiving treatment at our clinic, he and his family were back to adventuring. They've since traveled to Yellowstone National Park, Israel, and taken many other big trips.

This is why I treat every single person as a unique, one-of-a-kind case. Every person's tangled web of dysfunction is different and caused by a different combination of dysfunctional processes. The exam is how we open that cold-case file and start to uncover what's going on beneath the surface.

CHAPTER 13

OUR PROGRAM

THE PHASES OF DECLINE

The "phases of decline" refer to the stages someone struggling with chronic health problems will experience as their dysfunctional process advances. While this book is ultimately about hope and the encouragement that it is often possible to stop and reverse physical damage and disorders, you also need to take these phases of decline seriously because there is a point of no return. At this point, the body becomes so damaged that it's not possible to regenerate your health to a normal state. Let's take a look at the phases of decline for the three most common maladies I see in my clinic—brain disorders, knee pain, and neuropathy.

PHASES OF DECLINE FOR BRAIN DISORDERS

Phase One: Full Health

No symptoms expressed at all.

Phase Two: Easily Dismissible Symptoms

These are things like brain fog that just won't go away, difficulty focusing and concentrating for long periods of time, and a loss of attention to the things you normally enjoy and love. At this point, your brain cells are actually dying, yet most people won't take action, instead choosing to casually dismiss the changes. The patient usually doesn't take responsibility or action, at least not yet.

Phase Three/Four: Recognizable Symptoms

At this stage, things are beginning to progress. You may walk into a room and forget why you walked in there in the first place. Or you may call someone on the phone and forget why you called them. This is an advanced stage of brain degeneration. This is the point where the adult kids may tease their parents about having "old timers" syndrome or say things like "Mom is just losing it..." At this stage, it's very important to filter who you listen to. Your healthcare provider, your kids, your friends, or your spouse may laugh it off, but it's nothing to joke about. At this phase, you must stand up and take responsibility for your health. If you know something isn't right, keep pursuing a solution until you get answers.

Phase Five: The Limitation of Matter

At this stage, the brain is degenerated to the point where the person is no longer motivated and simply doesn't have the brain ability to solve their own problems. They no longer see themselves as the problem; instead, everyone else has a problem. When someone reaches this stage, it is very hard and nearly impossible to bring them back. It's a very serious case when someone gets to this stage. It's called "limitation of matter" because at this point, the brain has degenerated so far that it's unable to regenerate and repair to its former state. I don't accept patients for care who are at this stage of degeneration.

Common Treatments for Brain Disorders:

These are the common in-clinic treatments that I do for brain-based disorders.

- Clear Mind neurofeedback program - this tool instantly and non-invasively identifies brain dysfunction. I use these results to know which areas of the brain to stimulate to help it begin functioning optimally again.

- Exercise with oxygen therapy - This is simply putting an oxygen mask on the patient and having them ride a stationary bike for twenty minutes while breathing in pure oxygen.

- Hako-Med - This powerful machine helps stimulate proper nerve function.

- Pulse Electro-Magnetic Field (PEMF) machine - This machine is like a battery re-charger for your body. It helps to recharge the cells of the body to the perfect charge to maintain optimal cellular function.

- At-Home Exercises - Vagal stimulation exercises, 90 day brain and body detox, and proper nutritional supplementation.

PHASES OF DECLINE FOR KNEE PAIN

I classify chronic knee pain as anything that has existed for three months or longer. Most of the people who come see me for knee pain have had it for years, if not decades, and can barely walk or get out of a chair. They often have difficulty getting out of bed or off the couch, and their life is severely impacted by their pain. One of the first things I do with every knee pain patient is take x-rays of the knee. We can use regenerative medicine at the clinic, but in order for that treatment to be effective, there has to be a space between the knee joint as seen on the radiograph. The space is important because it means there is still tissue present that can be rehabilitated. If there's no space, they've reached the limitation of matter and have to be referred out for a knee replacement. I don't accept everyone that comes into the office as a patient. If I do the exam and, based on their results, I don't think I can help them, I refer the patient to a health professional who can better assist them.

However, if the x-ray shows enough spacing in the joint, I may start with a regenerative medicine treatment plan to help them eliminate their chronic pain and regain mobility. Here are some of the solutions that have worked exceptionally well for our knee pain patients.

Common Treatments for Knee Pain:

- The Ergo-Flex Knee-On-Track - This is a machine that decompresses the knee and opens up the joint space, promoting healing and pain relief.

- Oxygen therapy with exercise - I talked about this treatment earlier in the book, but this is simply putting an oxygen mask on the patient and having them ride a stationary bike for twenty minutes while breathing in oxygen.

- Hako-Med - This powerful machine helps stimulate proper nerve function.

- Laser therapy - This treatment decreases inflammation and pain by dilating the capillaries to promote blood flow and encourage the healing properties to access the joint.

- Pulse Electro-Magnetic Field (PEMF) machine - This machine is like a battery re-charger for your body. It helps to recharge the cells of the body to the perfect charge to maintain optimal cellular function.

- Trigenics - This modality activates the two main receptors of the brain so that they fire into the cerebellum, spinal cord and brain to decrease pain and increase mobility.

- The Ergo-Flex Knee-On-Track - This is a machine that decompresses the knee and opens up the joint space, promoting healing and pain relief.

PHASES OF DECLINE FOR NEUROPATHY:

Neuropathy patients are usually the most complicated cases because neuropathy can be caused by so many different dysfunctions. These patients often have oxygen problems, glucose problems, and their brain has deteriorated because of a lack of stimulation from their feet. Many people with neuropathy also have erectile or sexual dysfunction.

Phase One: The feet begin tingling or experiencing a pins and needles sensation.

Phase Two: Coldness and color changes in the toes and feet.
Phase Three: The tingling becomes a burning pain.
Phase Four: Loss of sensation in the legs, feet, toes.

Common Treatments for Neuropathy:

- Blood sugar regulation - I work with the patient to help them balance their blood sugar so their neurological system can stabilize and begin the work of healing.

- Spinal decompression - Many patients with neuropathy have L5 damage so I use decompression therapy to re-lieve the pressure on that area of the spine.

- Oxygen therapy with exercise - I talked about this treatment earlier in the book, but this is simply putting an oxygen mask on the patient and having them ride a stationary bike for twenty minutes while breathing in oxygen.

- Hako-Med on their feet - This powerful machine helps stimulate proper nerve function.

- Laser therapy - This treatment decreases inflammation and pain by dilating the capillaries to promote blood flow and encourage the healing properties to access the joint.

- Pulse Electro-Magnetic Field (PEMF) machine - This machine is like a battery re-charger for your body.

It helps to recharge the cells of the body to the perfect charge to maintain optimal cellular function.

- Trigenics - This modality activates the two main receptors of the brain so that they fire into the cerebellum, spinal cord and brain to decrease pain and increase mobility.

- Clear Mind neurofeedback program - this tool instantly and non-invasively identifies brain dysfunction. I use these results to know which areas of the brain to stimulate to help it start functioning optimally again.

- At-Home Exercises - Brain-Body-Gut 90 day detox and proper nutritional supplementation.

CUSTOM MADE

A truly custom, one-of-a-kind healthcare program will impact your health in a way you've never experienced before because it is created uniquely for you. I don't accept everyone for care. If someone isn't fully committed, they're too neurologically damaged, or they're too far degenerated, I'm not going to take them for care and waste their time or money. When I accept someone for care, I make them a promise that I'm on this journey with them, and we're in it to win it. I will exhaust every option I know in order to optimize their recovery. However, we both need to have realistic expectations. If their expectations are beyond what I can give them, we need to realign. I'm always going to under promise and over deliver, and sometimes tough love requires telling people the truth that they don't want to hear.

A custom healthcare program to heal your chronic disease always comes as a result of a thorough and effective neurological examination process, and it always addresses all aspects of your metabolic and neurological health. However, the truth is that if they don't follow the program I prescribe them, they're probably not going to get the results they want. No one is going to care more about your health than you. If you don't want to be well, live vibrantly, and leave a legacy, no one is going to do it for you. I'm totally committed to the patient, but they need to be "all in" too.

CHAPTER 14

A PERFECT PAIRING

I truly appreciate the opportunity to connect with you as a new patient and help you reconnect the damaged body systems to create a better life for yourself, your spouse, your children, their children, and for generations to come! How do you know I am the right chiropractor for you?

If you have experienced failures with traditional medicine, don't give up yet!

When you have been through experiences with traditional doctors that made you feel like there is nothing left to do, it is a good time to try working with a specially trained chiropractor. Nobody comes in with a mindset of being all-in and thoroughly committed, and that is okay. I felt that way when I had my first experience with a chiropractor.

If you know you need help, and you have been to a doctor who has not been able to get you to a place where you are feeling better, you may be at the point where you are wondering if something other than traditional medicine may be the right route for you.

I am happy to provide the education and create a program that will finally help you achieve the results you are looking for.

Do you have serious health concerns and want to feel better?

Just like me with my experiences as a marathon runner, I find that if you are at your wit's end with a health problem you are going to come to a functional neuro-metabolic chiropractor with an openness you may not have had previously.

You have been to a place where they took your insurance, but nothing changed for you in terms of your health and well-being. It may be time to invest in yourself and see where you are after our time together. It is less about the money and more about your mindset when it comes to making the changes that allow your body to heal itself.

Your family is behind you as part of your team.

In order to make the changes that will positively affect your life for the long haul, you need to have a support system outside of the office. It is much easier to make changes to your diet and exercise routines if there are family members who are willing to share the experience with you.

Your healing program is more than just you. It affects your spouse, your kids, and even your grandkids. Having honest and open conversations with them and getting them on board as part of your team helps you have accountability partners on your journey.

Your progress is an evolution.

We are here to engage you in a life-long healing system. There are no miracles here. If you are looking for healing within a week, we are probably not the right office for you. There must be a starting point and a goal to meet that occurs over three, six, or twelve months.

Once we understand what is happening in your body, I will give you options to meet your needs in a way that makes sense to you. Maybe you want a combination of things to do in the office and at home. Or maybe you want to focus on something that has been bothering you for a few weeks; or maybe there is something else that has been around for decades—or both. I am happy to give you my best recommendations to help you feel better.

There is usually more than one thing going on. It is usually worse than you thought and will take longer to get on a healing path!!

I am happy to meet you where you want to be healed. The better the communication between the two of us, the easier it becomes to create the treatment plan that works for you.

You have optimal health when your brain, GI tract and body work in concert. Everything is connected in a complex web of nerves, blood vessels, and tissues. If there is even a little bit of miscommunication between them, your health can be affected. They are all communicating with each other. You can think of these three pieces together as a computer network. It includes your spinal column, stomach, and your body. We look for places in the system where there is an area of malfunction that creates a warning sign with "blinky lights."

Maybe you have "blinky lights" in your brain. You see a specialist who looks primarily at those "blinky lights" and prescribes some medication to help turn them off. But then there are issues with your joints, so you go to an orthopedic surgeon. Then you have some stomach problems and go to a GI specialist. So, there are all these MD's working on you piece by piece.

Neuro-metabolic chiropractors look at all the "blinky lights" as a whole and connect the dots to determine the overall damage and how your body is affected in order to turn them off.

By having to go to the various specialists who are only working on one set of "blinky lights" at a time it may be hard to get answers to complex chronic health conditions. .

Your brain, body and GI tract must communicate perfectly for your optimal health. When they do not, health is lost. Typically, a doctor would treat the symptom. But we are here to look at all your systems and find the path to getting everything to work together for your greatest good. And when that happens, the symptoms lessen or disappear.

Do you want to live longer, reduce your risk of chronic diseases and/or dementia as you grow older, and have optimal days that make your life meaningful? Let us work together to bring joy back to your life. Your first step is to listen to that little voice telling you, "Now's the time. Let us do this." Go to our website at fairviewdc.com to ask any questions or schedule an appointment.

It is common to see patients that have been everywhere looking for help with complex chronic health conditions. They have "blinky lights" on various parts of their bodies. Traditional diagnosing focuses on just the condition being evaluated and not on the big picture. We try to look at the big picture and connect the dots to complex health conditions. The chart below illustrates typical "blinky light" symptoms when we first meet someone. Can you find anything on the chart that you are experiencing? Did you circle things under the body, brain, and GI functions? Did you circle a lot of them? Have you been to a lot of doctors already?

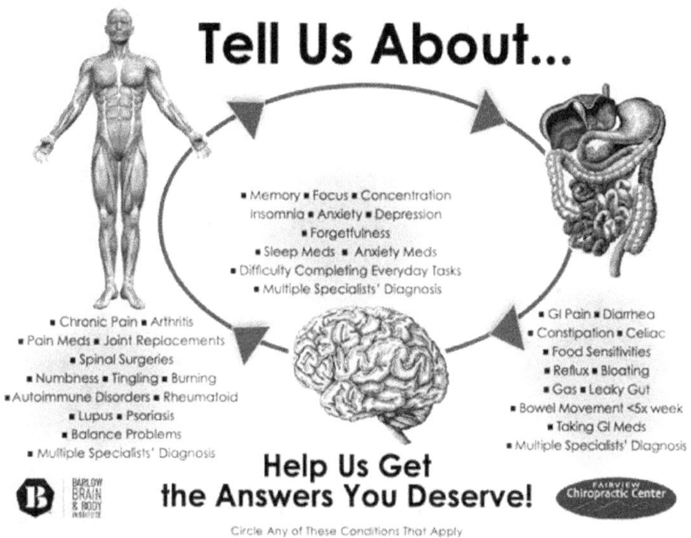

I'll close with this idea: We all have "blinky lights" in our lives that can be identified and optimized to improve our health and the quality of our lives. If you have been searching for answers to complex chronic health conditions and are still looking for help, consider seeing a doctor who has been trained to read the body's own signals, do the types of testing required, and have treatment and lifestyle changes that allow you to live your best life.

Where Are Your Blinky Lights?

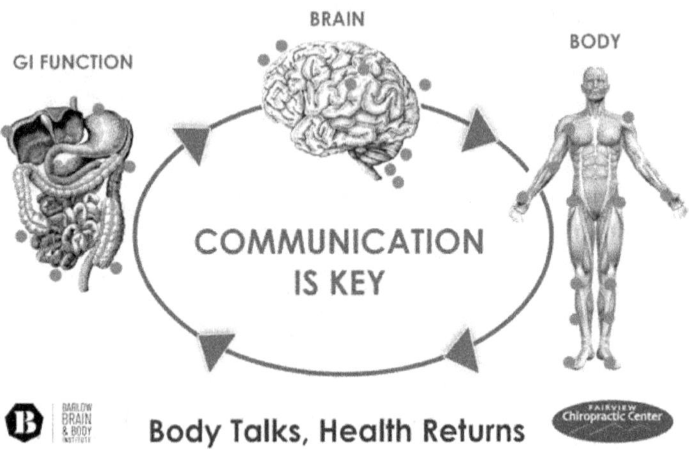

**Let us help by finding the "blinky lights"
that are affecting your health!**

ABOUT THE AUTHOR

A New Jersey native, Dr. Reilly (Edward G. Reilly BA,MBA, DC, CCSP,FIAMI,KDT-C, GT-C0 had a successful career with a Fortune 500 company, managing a team of 50 employees and traveling the country. However, he repeatedly felt a calling to a different life and career, although he was initially unsure exactly what he was being called to do. Two extremely dramatic and positive experiences in a chiropractic office lead him to believe that the life of a healer was his true vocation. He quit his job, sold all his possessions, and moved to Georgia to attend Life University of Chiropractic. He graduated with honors in 1996, and opened his practice in Fairview, NC in 1998.

Since that time, Dr. Reilly has dedicated himself to providing not only the finest traditional chiropractic care but also providing his patients with the very latest in cutting edge technology so that they might experience optimum healing and symptom relief. To that end, he has completed an additional 4,000 hours of post-doctoral training in medicine. He offers, and is certified in, therapies such as Graston Therapy, LiteCure Class 4 Laser therapy, Trigenics, Advanced Functional Neurology, Spinal Decompression Traction, and PEMF NRG therapy. Many of these therapies are found primarily in pro sports team locker rooms—but you too can receive the same treatment as a top NFL player in Dr. Reilly's office. Dr. Reilly has delivered over 1.000 health lectures, including being selected to speak at the last 2 international conferences on PEMF and neuropathy. He was President of the NC Chiropractic Association in 2013, and was named Doctor of the Year by the organization that year.

Dr. Reilly has two children, Connor, a sophomore engineering major at UNCC, and Leia, a high school senior and aspiring flutist. As an avid runner, cyclist, and hiker, Dr. Reilly understands – and strives to educate his patients on – the role exercise and proper nutrition play in achieving optimal health. He has been an Associate of the International Foundation for Nutrition and Health since 1999 and offers the latest in supplements and exercise devices, such as the Posture Pulley.

Dr. Reilly's caring spirit extends beyond his practice. Active in the community, he sponsors many nonprofit organizations, is an active volunteer for many others, and sits on the board of Food for Fairview, a local food pantry. He serves as team chiropractor for the AC Reynolds High School football team. In addition, he participates in many community organizations, such as the Fairview Business Association.

TESTIMONIALS OF HEALING

"I was unable to stand or walk more than a few feet because I had severe pain in my shoulders. Within a week of treatment the pain had subsided. I would like to personally tell you that suffering is unnecessary. Within a week the pain was gone, it's a miracle. I'd invite anyone to call me for my recommendation to Fairview Chiropractic Center."

—LINN R.

"I have been struggling the past two years with pain in my lower leg and foot. I have been out of all impact activities for the past ten months without help from drugs or physical therapy. A bone scan could not find my problem. Now through chiropractic care I am back on my feet literally. Visit a chiropractor; drugs are not always the answer."

—MELISSA G.

"I had a sore neck and couldn't turn my head left or right. My ring finger and little finger were numb even though I had two surgeries on it two years earlier to correct it. Now I have no neck pain and the numbness in my fingers is gone. Do not have surgery until you try chiropractic care. I had the surgery and was not much different."

—JAMES B.

"I had carpal tunnel syndrome, sacroiliac and hip joint problems for months. I tried physical and occupational therapies, drugs and other chiropractors without much success. Dr Reilly's approach is very gentle and chiropractic care has prevented me from having carpal tunnel surgery."

—KK

"I had low back pain and headaches for years that had recently gotten worse. I took muscle relaxants and pain relievers. Today I have no more low back pain or headaches. This is the best and most cost effective way to solve these kinds of problems."

—CINDY G.

"I was experiencing severe neck and back pain for one month. I was diagnosed with a herniated cervical disc by two neurosurgeons. They both recommended surgery to correct my problem. After several treatments in Dr Reilly's office my problem was corrected. The treatment I received was beyond my expectations. I would highly recommend Fairview Chiropractic as an alternative to surgery."

—LARRY L.

"I had pain in my left hip for 20 years and tingling in my toes for a year. In two weeks my hip was fixed and my toes were better. See Dr Ed."

—ROGER G.L.

"I had low back and right leg pain, neck and shoulder, arm and hand pain and tingling for over four years. I tried physical therapy on my back and leg. After several treatments my pain is almost gone, I feel like a new person, it feels so good not to have that hot burning pain. Get help soon, it really helps, I am so glad I did."

—EDITH F.

"I live in South Carolina. I injured my hand and couldn't perform my work as a drafter. Several MDs suggested surgery to correct my problem. A friend referred me to your office. After three visits my wrist and hand pain were gone and I could go back to work. I would encourage anyone with wrist or hand pain to consult with DR Reilly. Thank You."

—ELKE G.

"My baby cried constantly from birth until about six weeks ago when I took Jonah to see Dr Reilly. After one treatment, Dr Reilly gently touched my baby's neck with his index finger and my baby immediately stopped crying right in my arms. Now my baby is happy and hardly ever cries. It made a world of difference, it's like he's a whole new baby."

—DD

"I would like to thank Dr. Reilly so much for introducing me to Neurofeedback. In the last month it has helped me tremendously with my focus, my sleep and most of all it has given me an overall sense of well being and calm. Things that used to bother me roll of my back"now. I would recommend this to everyone!"

—JEANETTE R.

"I started coming to Dr. Ed's office two years ago for chronic headaches. Within the first week, my headaches were gone. After a year, Dr. Ed told me he could help my four-year-old daughter with her chronic ear infection. I started bringing Laura in and, sure enough, within a few months later her ear infection started to decrease. By the end of the cold season, she no longer had ear trouble. After seeing the great results with my daughter, I decided to bring my nephew, Nathaniel, who had two rounds of tubes in his ear and they (the doctors) were talking for a third time. I brought him in and sure enough, Dr. Ed went right to work and Nathaniel is ear trouble free. Now I bring all four kids and we have had no colds or ear trouble since. And if we get a cold, it's gone within days. Thank you Dr. Ed and staff for taking care of my family."

—MISTIE

"I had a long history of knee problems, which included having to get shots in both knees every three months and dealing with radiating pain from my hip to my ankles on a daily basis. I took pain pills every day, three times a day, and had two arthroscopic surgeries. The next thing was to have a full or partial knee replacement. My wife was coming to Dr. Reilly for her knee problems. I came with her on visits and had questions for the doctor. Dr. Reilly took the time to talk with me. I was pleased with our conversation and set up an appointment to get started. The first thing was to have x-rays. When that was complete, we talked about what he could do to help me out. With heat and traction on my back and neurolumen (advanced laser therapy), it began to work. But what really helped was the Graston therapy (advanced myofascial release – used by pro sports teams). It seemed to work overnight.

I started the ChiroThin Weight Loss program to help remove weight, help relieve stress from my joints and give me a better lifestyle. I am happy to say – IT REALLY WORKS!

I am so glad that I came to Fairview Chiropractic Center and Dr. Reilly. I can now walk better and long with little or no pain. I have seen my orthopedic doctor and we have put off my knee replacement and I have not had shots in my knees in over 5 months. I take pain medication very seldom now. Dr. Reilly has given me hope that I will not have a knee replacement in the near future.

A BIG THANKS TO DR. REILLY AND HIS STAFFF!!! They made me feel as if I was a part of their family."

—FORREST R.

"I am being treated for Spinal Stenosis. Before coming to see Dr. Reilly I had injections to eliminate the pain for 3 months or more. They did not work. Surgery was mentioned but I wasn't ready for the long surgery and lengthy recovery.

I saw an article for in the newspaper about what Dr. Reilly could do for stenosis so I called for an Appointment. After a round of treatment: laser therapy, traction, magnetic resonance therapy and heat therapy, weekly for several months my pain was gone. I had 2 years mostly pain free with just one set back. After a month of weekly treatments, I am once again on a once a month regimen of traction and adjustment plus my daily exercises.

Thank you Dr. Reilly!"

—MARY R.

"I had suffered with dull low back pain for years. The week prior to coming to Fairview Chiropractic Center, the lower back pain when I was lying down was moderate and was I couldn't lift my left leg, stand straight and walking was very difficult. I did not seek any other treatments before coming to Dr. Reilly. In addition to my low back pain, I have always had a sore neck. Since treatment I have had a full range of motion. Dr. Reilly and his staff have been wonderful. Everything from paperwork to machines and exercises were explained in great detail. This was my first experience with chiropractic care. I am amazed at how many health issues can be addressed with chiropractic care. I would highly recommend Fairview Chiropractic Center and Dr. Reilly."

—JENNIFER A.

"Last fall my family physician ordered an MRI of my back. When the results came back she referred me to a spine surgeon. He recommended a 4 to 4 1/2 hour surgery to repair a herniated disc and remove bone spurs, and then he would fuse the bone fragments to build up my back then place rods to hold everything in place. I chose not to have surgery so I have continued to suffer severe back pain with neuropathy down both legs, worsening for the last six to eight months.In June of this year God allowed and blessed me to learn of Dr. Reilly and his Chiropractic Center. Immediately made an appointment to find out if he could help me. When I saw Dr. Reilly, after x-rays and examination, told me he could help me and gave me a 70-100% chance to be helped without surgery. I began treatment of realignment, laser therapy, traction, heat treatment and MagneticResonance Therapy, which is amazing.All these treatments have given me my life back. I am now smiling, feeling much better and able to enjoy life again. It is a joy to arise in the morning knowing a much better day is ahead, whereas it was hard to face each day, even with pain medication that did not give me much relief. I thank God everyday for Dr. Reilly and his wonderful staff. I also want to thank my wonderful husband for driving me to my appointments and patiently waiting for me to have my treatments."

—REBECCA B.

"I came to Fairview Chiropractic Center and Dr. Reilly with severe pain in the left side of my lower back. The pain started after I had spent several hours on the computer in an awkward position. For the pain I took too much pain killer, which resulted in an intestinal bleed. I was hospitalized and in ICU for that. I complained of the back pain and they took an x-ray in the hospital and it showed arthritis. Again, pain medications were prescribed, however They only helped temporarily and after my ICU stay I was looking for an alternative.

Dr. Reilly was highly recommended to me. I made my first appointment with the Fairview Chiropractic Center to hear Dr. Reilly's diagnosis and to learn what his plan for me would be. His choice of procedure and scheduling has improved my condition Considerably. I would tell others to choose a chiropractor very carefully, as I did. I would most definitely recommend the Fairview Chiropractic Center with its professional staff."

—ERWIN B.

"I came to Dr. Reilly because I could not sit and I could hardly walk because of the pain down my leg. I had the problem about a month before I came and did not seek any other care. I feel like a new person after completion of my treatment plan. I have no pain and I am back to doing everything I could do before. Overall, I feel better physically. I would tell others to please try this so you can avoid surgery like did."

—BERNICE K.

"I was having balance problems when I was doing water aerobics. I realized that I did not having any feeling in my feet and could not stand on one foot for very long at all. I knew my feet did not have much feeling in them for a long time due to diabetes, but I did not realize how bad it had gotten. Thinking back, I would say over the last two years, I had been losing feeling in my feet. If I touched my feet with my hand or put my foot on my leg it was ice cold, but I could never tell that they were cold. I told my Medical Doctor about my feet but he never suggested any treatment. The LiteCure laser treatment and the Rebuilder foot bath that Dr. Reilly recommendations have made a big difference in my life. My toes now have a pink color instead of looking gray. My feet are not ice cold anymore when I touch them. When my feet get cold I can feel it now. I am anxious to see if This continues after my treatments are completed. I have told some co-workers how much this has helped me. One of my friends is going to see a Podiatrist that her Medical Doctor referred her to, she is also a diabetic, I suggested that she go to Fairview Chiropractic Center and consult with Dr. Reilly."

—DENISE T.

"I first began seeing Dr. Reilly in June 2007. I first injured my back 10 years ago while I was working at a fast food restaurant. I saw a chiropractor then for several months and was diagnosed with a herniated disc. The pain was almost constant and got so bad that I was unable to dress myself, take a shower myself or even put my own shoes on. The chiropractor that I was seeing then was unable to provide any relief. The pain continued to get worse and I had to take a leave of absence from work. Eventually, with several months of bed rest, the pain subsided and I was able to return to work. In the back of my mind, I was always worried that I would re-injure the same spot. Once I began working as a nurse, the constant pulling and tugging began to aggravate the old injury again. So in June 2007 I began to see Dr. Reilly to see if I could get some relief from the pain. I had the usual adjustments at first, followed by cold therapy and DTS (spinal traction). After the very first week of visits I already felt some relief. I believe the traction was what made the biggest difference. I have only been able to keep working because of Dr. Reilly. I still see him for regular adjustments and have told everyone that he is the real deal!!! I literally am only able to continue working because of him. No-one should ever doubt the power of true chiropractic to relieve pain and restore function."

—RACHEL R., RN

"I was referred to Dr. Reilly by my brother who is a longtime patient of Fairview Chiropractic Center. I had a 'pinched nerve' in my low back for about a month and was taking advil for it on

on a daily basis. After completing my treatment plan I was pain free and felt that my spine was straight and that my whole back was treated and is better."

—SHERRY S.

"I just want to say thank you to so much to everyone at Fairview Chiropractic for making me feel so great! The pain I was experiencing before I began chiropractic care was very intense and left I am miserable. I was unable to find relief with my medical doctor and decided to give chiropractic care is a try. I was suffering from a sciatic nerve problem and a bulging disc. My the sciatic nerve problem was a nerve problem at all; it was an alignment problem. My right hip was so out of alignment that it was pulling on everything. After Dr. Reilly adjusted me a few times my pain was completely gone and hasn't ever come back! I suffered needlessly for years. Then I injured myself and as a result had a bulging disc. Most times this requires surgery to repair but Dr. Reilly suggested I try traction on the DTS machine. After 3 visits I could really tell a difference and with a few more I was once again pain free - without surgery! I really can't say enough about the care and help I have received from Fairview Chiropractic!"

—JESSICA H.

"How could I have imagined what was in store for me the morning I got out of bed noticing a slight discomfort in my left buttock. Over the course of the day it didn't go away as I had hoped, but also seemed no worse so I didn't dwell on it. Thinking I had slept in some position to bring it on, I hoped the next night's rest would make it go away. The second morning, the discomfort was more distinct, with slight pain down my leg so I decided to see the Chiropractor who has helped me with previous back pain problems. Dr Reilly did an assessment through various bending, stretching and reaching exercises and said the problem was not in my leg but in my lower back, (L-5 disc) which is fairly common and treatable. I began regular chiropractic treatments including electro-stimulations and adjustments, later adding decompression traction. The pain down my leg progressed steadily as a particular nerve became severely infected. Sitting was nearly impossible leading Dr. Reilly to do an x-ray which showed a more difficult problem with the disc. He advised me to see my family doctor. Along with continued chiropractic treatments including now a cold laser, my family physician ordered pain medications and an MRI. We decided the problem could be corrected without surgery, so we reached out to a Carolina Spine specialist for further expertise. With epidural steroid injections and on-going chiropractic work, this team approach has been very beneficial and I am feeling almost 'all the way back.' I commend Dr. Reilly for his warm, caring professional work throughout. It is fortunate for people in Fairview area that we can partake of his services and rely on his expert advice."

—FRED B.

"I would recommend anyone with a back problem to Dr. Reilly."

—MARK P.

"I had been suffering with lower back pain and numbness in my right calf for about 2 years. I read about Dr. Reilly and Fairview Chiropractic Center in an ad and decided to give chiropractic a try. I had already done the medical treatments of prescription drugs, injections and physical therapy and it did not help relieve my pain. Upon completing the treatment regimen Dr. Reilly recommended, my back pain is all but gone and I no longer have any numbness in my calf. I can now do anything I want without experiencing pain. I have recommended many people with back problems to Dr. Reilly, it's definitely worth trying."

—VICKI L.

"I was experiencing lower back pain due to a compressed nerve at L5. I was having severe pain down my right leg that had persisted for two weeks and was not getting better. I started to take Advil for the pain prior to coming to Fairview Chiropractic Center. Dr. Reilly evaluated me and prescribed a course of treatment to remedy my problem. The treatment consisted of decompression traction and spinal adjustments that were precise through the course of treatment and corrected my problem. In addition to my pain when I was gone my movements became more fluid and I experienced weight loss. I will strongly encourage anyone I know experiencing structural problems to seek help. At Fairview Chiropractic Center to alleviate their problems."

—PAUL H.

"I am a long time patient of Dr. Reilly's. In the past I have come in when I had a problem and after I was pain free I didn't come in again until I was in pain. I never followed Dr. Reilly's recommendation for maintenance care. That is until this last episode: I was carried into Dr. Reilly's office on 11/19/12 after lifting a heavy bale of hay. I could not walk for anything. Dr. Reilly was very concerned and sent me to the emergency room for evaluation. All they did there was give me pain medications and send me home with the recommendation to see a neurosurgeon. 10 days later I was finally able to get an MRI that confirmed Dr. Reilly's suspicions that I had a serious herniated disc. All the medical doctor could recommend was steroid injection and surgery – the sooner the better. Dr. Reilly had a different idea – give his treatment a chance. I followed his treatment plan to the tee. I had the decompression traction with chiropractic adjustments regularly. Within 10 days I was seeing results. I was able to sleep through the night without waking because of pain. The pain was reduced by 60%. By the time I saw the neurosurgeon on 1/9/13 I was pain free. They offered another injection that I refused, she couldn't believe I was in no pain without surgery and she didn't want to hear what had helped either. As of today I have been released to maintenance care and you can believe me when I say I will stick to it this time! My advice to anyone seeing Dr. Reilly and his wonderful staff – when you improve and are told to follow up once a month – DO IT!"

—RONNIE W.

"I came to Dr. Reilly as a 58-year-old with severe pain in both arms from pressure on the nerves in my neck that was the result of three whiplash-type neck injuries, poor posture, and forward head thrust from sitting at a computer eight-plus hours a day for seven years. The pain was so bad that, at times, I could barely raise my hand to rub my My nose, I was unable to lift anything, driving my car had me in tears and a solid night's sleep. Thinking that the pain was just caused by loading the U-haul by myself for my recent move from the west coast, rearranging furniture in the house and stacking a cord of firewood, I suffered for four months before seeking help. Coming to Dr. Reilly has been my first experience in Chiropractic care. I prefer natural remedies whenever possible and I certainly didn't want to even considered the possibility of surgery to relieve my pain. At my initial consultation, Dr. Reilly outlined a multi-phase treatment plan that initially would include treatments and adjustments and eventually would add exercise therapy to strengthen the muscles. He explained that much of the results would depend on how willing I was to actively participate in my own road to wellness. Within a month of the beginning of my treatment the pain was significantly reduced and continued to diminish with each visit. After 2 months the pain was gone, I had full motion in both arms, I was gaining back the strength in my arms, and was finally able to sleep comfortably through the night without waking up frequently from the discomfort. In less than six months I have gone from the initial three visits a week that were needed to deal with the immediate problem of the pain, to coming in once a month for an adjustment. I have gone from the desperate need for relief from pain to working on total wellness with exercises that are designed to strengthen the muscles and prevent or off set future problems. I sincerely appreciate Dr. Reilly's honesty in his evaluation of my conditions and the treatment plan to treat the causes and not just the symptoms. I also appreciate the delightfully friendly, professional and efficient staff for treating me as a person and not just as a name on the appointment calendar. I feel gently cared for at every level. The efficiency of this office is impressive. There is not the "usual" long waiting periods that I've experienced at other medical offices, yet I never feel like I'm being rushed when I come in for a visit. I am truly impressed with the care I've received and would highly recommend Fairview Chiropractic Center to anyone looking for chiropractic care."

—CAROLYN M.

"I came to Dr. Reilly's office the end of March. I was very nervous and leery. I had heard all of the "old wives' tales" about chiropractors. How all they wanted is your money and that most of them were quacks. My family doctor referred me to him. I was having a lot of pain in my shoulder and numbness in my arm. I have had an MRI done. I have three bulging discs in my neck. My doctor told me he would advise me to see a chiropractor. My next option was to see a surgeon. This wasn't the first time I was told I ought to consider a chiropractor. I'm on disability. I suffer from fibromyalgia and thoracic outlet syndrome. I have gone through years of therapy. I'm on a limited income. All I could think about was the rumors I had heard about chiropractors. All they wanted was to "crack your back" and charge outrageous prices.

Well, I went home with Dr. Reilly's phone number in my hand with another pain medicine prescription. I started to throw it away. I finally broke down and thought what the heck, I'd been through a lot worse. This was the second time I had been told I should think about seeing a chiropractor. That was one call I'll never regret making. Dr. Reilly's staff is as precious as he is wonderful. Dr. Reilly is a life savior. He has helped me so much. He saw how much pain I was in. He's never been excited about money. He understood my situation from the first day. He has helped me so much. I don't know where I'd be right now or what kind of shape I'd be in now if I hadn't made that phone call. I would recommend him to anyone. He's the type of doctor that if he can't help you he'll try to find someone who can. Dr. Reilly is a God send. His staff is just so caring also.

—TERRY M.

www.ingramcontent.com/pod-product-compliance
Lightning Source LLC
Chambersburg PA
CBHW071021260726

48662CB00023B/1262